Praise for *Holy Sex!* . . .

"Some books are worth reading because they make an important point, others for the sheer delight of the writing. Greg Popcak's *Holy Sex!* is both. Wherever one stands on the fine points of Catholic teaching about sex, Popcak reveals its deeply sensual core, debunking popular stereotypes of Catholicism as somehow anti-erotic. Think of this book as Thomas Aquinas meets Dr. Ruth, and enjoy!"

> — JOHN L. ALLEN JR., Senior Correspondent for
> the *National Catholic Reporter* and author of
> *Mega-Trends in Catholicism: Ten Forces Turning
> the Catholic Church Upside Down* (Doubleday).

"Dynamic, faithful, funny, and informative, *Holy Sex!* demonstrates how the Truth will set you free. Popcak offers a path to authentic 'sexual liberation' — not the bondage to libido that passes for freedom in our culture, but the freedom to love. Combining practical wisdom with the wisdom of the ages, Popcak leads men and women to the love they long for. *Holy Sex!* deserves a big Amen!"

> — CHRISTOPHER WEST, Fellow, Theology of the Body Institute;
> Author, *The Love That Satisfies: Reflections on Eros and Agape*

"Though this may shock much of the churchgoing world, 'purity' and 'prude' are not synonymous terms. This witty, well-researched book provides some much needed insight concerning God's design for married sexuality. As an Evangelical reader I was particularly interested in Popcak's intelligent, thought-provoking challenge to the carte-blanche acceptance of birth control by the church at large. Couples — be they Catholic, Evangelical, or otherwise — would do well to consider Popcak's challenge to rethink the sexual status quo."

> — ED GUNGOR, Lead Pastor of the People's Church in Tulsa,
> Author of *There's More to the Secret* and *The Vow*

"In this invigorating, informative, eye-opening book, Dr. Greg Popcak reveals the pristine beauty of God's original plan for sex. For those who think that shallow eroticism or joyless, mechanical intercourse are the only two options for one's sex life, Dr. Popcak invites you to think again. With upbeat prose and practical examples, Dr. Popcak takes up Pope John Paul's Theology of the Body and lays out a whole new way of thinking about sex — God's way."

> — FATHER THOMAS D. WILLIAMS, L.C., Dean of Theology at
> Regina Apostolorum University (Rome), Vatican Analyst for
> CBS News, and author of *Spiritual Progress: Becoming the Christian*
> *You Want to Be* and *Greater Than You Think:*
> *A Theologian Answers the Atheists about* God

"It is no surprise to see Dr. Popcak treat marital sex as a truly joyful thing in *Holy Sex!* As he so clearly points out, God designed man and woman to communicate his love in their spiritual and physical union. If married couples could actually experience their lovemaking as an expression of God's creative, joyous and renewing love, wow!"

> — MOST REV. R. DANIEL CONLON, Bishop of Steubenville, Ohio

"I can safely guarantee that all who read this book will find something new and helpful, will laugh a lot, and may even be shocked at what Dr. Popcak reveals to be compatible with Catholic teaching. Clearly, Dr. Popcak is a chaste, faithful, learned Catholic man with mountains of experience working with couples. I have been waiting a long time for someone like him to write a book like this. I am confident that spouses who follow his advice will become holier and better partners. Those who are holier are certainly better lovers and thanks to *Holy Sex!* we now know the many ways this is true. Great book!"

> — JANET E. SMITH, Father Michael J. McGivney Chair
> of Life Ethics, Sacred Heart Major Seminary, Detroit

"Looking at contemporary popular culture, one finds that sex is overrated and undervalued. Greg Popcak's fine book helps to set things straight on both counts. He explains with intelligence and humor what some have learned only through painful experience, and many have still not learned, namely, that the joy of sex is not to be found in 'liberation' from moral principles, but in its unique power to unite a man and woman as faithful partners in the love-building and life-giving union that marriage is."

— ROBERT P. GEORGE, McCormick Professor of Jurisprudence
and Director of the James Madison Program
in American Ideals and Institutions, Princeton University

"*Holy Sex!* is the book that all Catholic young adults have been waiting for. Popcak uses both scientific references and Catholic tradition to put forth a sexual theology that is both relevant and faithful to tradition."

— MIKE HAYES, author of *Googling God* and
Managing Editor of BustedHalo.com

"Greg Popcak is a wise and funny guy. He combines the ancient wisdom of the Faith with the best that contemporary science and compassionate human understanding have to offer in warm, generous, and practical insights that have already been invaluable to thousands. This book will only add to that rich legacy."

— MARK P. SHEA, Senior Content Editor, CatholicExchange.com

"Few people can successfully mix humor with a thought-provoking look at the depth of the Catholic faith on love and marriage. But Greg Popcak has managed to do just that in his exceptional book *Holy Sex!* This should be on the bookshelf of every engaged and married couple — after they've read it of course!"

— ANDY ALDERSON, Executive Director of
the Couple to Couple League

"In the last four decades, too many Americans have been led astray by self-styled experts promising sexual liberation and happiness, only to end up with broken hearts and broken bodies. By combining theological insight and psychological wisdom, Dr. Gregory Popcak offers a different path to men and women looking for a way to find happiness and virtue in their sexual lives. *Holy Sex!* is a powerful guide for navigating the joys and sorrows of sex."

— W. BRADFORD WILCOX, Director of the Marriage Matters Project
and Assistant Professor of Sociology at the University of Virginia

HOLY
Sex!

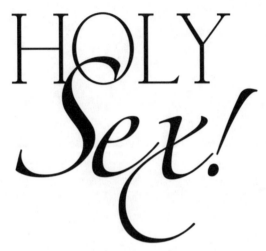

HOLY *Sex!*

A CATHOLIC GUIDE TO TOE-CURLING, MIND-BLOWING, INFALLIBLE LOVING

GREGORY K. POPCAK, PH.D.

A Crossroad Book
The Crossroad Publishing Company
New York

The Crossroad Publishing Company
16 Penn Plaza – 481 Eighth Avenue, Suite 1550
New York, NY 10001

Printed in the United States of America on acid-free paper

The text of this book is set in 11/16 Goudy Old Style.
The display faces are Zapfino and Sackers Light Classic Roman.

Library of Congress Cataloging-in-Publication Data

Popcak, Gregory K.
    Holy sex! : a Catholic guide to toe-curling, mind-blowing, fallible loving / Gregory K. Popcak.
       p. cm.
    ISBN-13: 978-0-8245-2471-5 (alk. paper)
    ISBN-10: 0-8245-2471-3 (alk. paper)
    1. Sex – Religious aspects – Catholic Church. 2. Catholic Church – Doctrines. I. Title.
BX1795.S48P66 2008
241'.66 – dc22   2007051315

1   2   3   4   5   6   7   8   9   10   12   11   10   09   08

CONTENTS

Quizzes

Exercises

PART ONE

Christianity's Best-Kept Secret

A fruitful kiss, this, and wonderful for its astounding kindness, which does not press mouth to mouth but unites God with humanity.
> — St. Bernard of Clairvaux, *On the Song of Songs*

AN INTRODUCTION TO HOLY SEX

You are about to discover Christianity's best kept secret: the mystical power of sexual love and the surprising, practical insights this tradition reveals to enable you and your beloved to "rise in ecstasy toward the Divine."*

In *Holy Sex!* you will discover what it takes to celebrate a toe-curling, eye-popping, mind-blowing, deeply spiritual, and profoundly sacramental sexuality — a sexual relationship that is both fully sensual and fully equipped to move beyond sensuality so that it can become an authentically transformative, spiritual encounter. Heaven will be wedded to earth as you and your spouse walk the path toward becoming Infallible Lovers, the kind of lovers who can infuse their marital lives with a passion that reaches biblical proportions. Literally.

---

*Pope Benedict XVI, *Deus Caritas Est.*

If these sound like big promises, they are meant to be. By the end of this book, you and your beloved will know how to create a passion that will make the angels smile and the neighbors sick with jealousy.

SURPRISING INSIGHTS FROM TRADITION

Most people believe the lie that Christians, and Catholic Christians in particular, have a dim, ignorant, and pleasure-killing view of sex. Nothing could be further from the truth. Not only *can* faithful Christian couples experience a sexual life that could make even the most jaded pagan jealous. Even more remarkably, Christian lovers are virtually *commanded* by God and their faith to do so. If this comes as a surprise to you, you're not alone. Most couples have bought into the lies that keep them from their passionate inheritance. Most people think that only secular sexperts or ancient, moldering pagan mystics have anything to teach the world about sex. Most people have never encountered the truth, the beauty, the goodness, and the vitality that is the mystical Christian spirituality of sex or the practical wisdom it imparts to those couples willing to seek it. Now you can know the truth, and the truth will set your love free.

In my capacity as a talk radio psychotherapist and author of several books on marriage and family life, I'm regularly invited to give workshops on sex and marriage. I have shared many of the principles revealed in this book with audiences across the country. Here are some examples of the feedback I've gotten from my encounters with couples.

"Why didn't anyone tell me this before? You really opened my eyes. Thank you for showing us what marital love could be and giving us the tools to make it happen." — *Erin, Buffalo, New York*

"I've been around, and I thought I knew everything about sex. I came away from your talk stunned. I hadn't begun to scratch the surface before today. I'm ashamed to admit that my wife had to drag me to your talk. I'm so glad she did. This is the best thing that ever happened to our marriage."

— *Jim, Dallas, Texas*

"Before I heard you, I thought good Christians were supposed to be ashamed of their sexuality. Thank you for showing me the truth. I can't wait to put your suggestions into practice. My husband isn't going to know what hit him!"
— Renee, Ann Arbor, Michigan

"This was wonderful. Faithful and practical! We're going to remember this as the weekend that changed our marriage. I've been married thirty years, but you opened up a whole new world for us." — Matt, Chicago, Illinois

What are these people — and thousands of others like them — responding to? The truth, the whole truth, and nothing but the truth about Holy Sex. Perhaps you are someone who believes that Christians know nothing worth knowing about sex — except how *not* to have fun while you "do it." Or perhaps you're someone (Christian or not) who believes that sex is "good," but, at best, a "nice thing to do at the end of the day if you have the time and energy." Either way, you're in for the shock of your life. This book not only explodes those myths and many others. It helps you mine the depths of a tradition that reveals the intimate core of sexuality and enables you to encounter lovemaking as God created it to be experienced — as a fully passionate, totally sensual, completely spiritual, remarkably transformational, revelatory, incarnational relationship. Consider this book your invitation to become the lover God wants you to be.

WHAT'S IN THIS BOOK?

Part One of *Holy Sex!* blows apart the lies you've been told about Christianity and sex and introduces you to the freeing truths of Infallible Loving. You'll come to view sex as a microcosm of your entire relationship. You'll discover what it takes to experience the kind of passion that challenges you and your mate to become better lovers and better people.

Part Two gives you the tools to tap into the Five Powers of Holy Sex. You'll discover how to expand your capacity to celebrate the *sacred, redemptive, heavenly, uniting,* and *creative* nature of sacred loving. You'll learn to experience sex as a transformative encounter with incarnational love that unites God himself with you and your beloved.

Part Three gives you everything you need to apply the principles of *Holy Sex!* to your marriage. You'll encounter many tips and techniques you and your spouse can use to become Infallible Lovers, capable of creating an authentic sexual relationship rooted in deep intimacy, soulful sensuality, and a vision that propels you toward perfection in love.

Finally, Part Four offers the practical guidance you need to overcome common sexual problems and obstacles that threaten your ability to experience everything your marriage was meant to be.

HOLY SEX: CAN YOU HANDLE IT?

In my work as the founder and executive director of the Pastoral Solutions Institute, I both conduct and supervise literally thousands of hours of pastoral tele-counseling every year with a predominantly Catholic population. People from around the world contact the Institute looking for faith-filled answers to life's difficult questions. In my direct work with clients, I've had the opportunity to help countless people work through painful marriages and difficult sexual problems in frank and faithful discussions. I've also coached innumerable couples in solid relationships who wanted to take things to the next level. I have had the privilege of guiding these couples to a place of greater peace, joy, intimacy, and passion. In the course of our sessions, they have discovered what you are about to learn: wherever you have been, whatever you have experienced, and regardless of where you are, God has an abundant banquet of love in store for you.

Some couples sneer at the idea that Holy Sex can be a path to authentic marital happiness. Instead of nurturing the Tree of Love and waiting to eat, at the peak of ripeness, the abundant fruit their effort produces, some people would rather spare themselves the effort, ignore the tree, and simply eat whatever fruit happens to fall to the ground, settling for what is cheap, easy, and often rotten.

God offers the joys of Holy Sex to everyone. Unfortunately, not everyone thinks Holy Sex is for them. But if you're willing to open your mind to the reality that there *is* more for you and your beloved, and if you're willing to commit to the labor that real love requires, then I am confident that you'll discover that Holy Sex is for you.

Can you handle the truth? Turn the page and find out.

1 SEX, LIES, AND THE REAL THING

God who created man out of love also calls him to love — the fundamental and innate vocation of every human being. For man is created in the image and likeness of God who is himself love. **Since God created him man and woman, their mutual love becomes an image of the absolute and unfailing love with which God loves man. It is good, very good, in the Creator's eyes.** — Catechism of the Catholic Church no. 1604; emphasis added

Walk into any bookstore and you'll find its shelves are positively pregnant with books about sex. Thanks to texts on tantric sex, karmic sex, kosher sex, sex for one, sex for several, and sexy sex for sex's sake, our culture has advanced to the point where you can do it on a plane, you can do it on a train, you can do it here, or there. Yes, my friends, you can do it anywhere — with confidence, impunity, and even, if you are so inclined, with malice aforethought.

But in the midst of the sea of information about sex, the unanswered question is "Can you do it . . . as a Christian?" To which the cynic responds, "Of course not!" And this goes double if you happen to be a Catholic Christian, in which case, the cynic would answer, "Not only can you not do it, you should be ashamed of yourself for even thinking about it."

The cynics are wrong.

Uber-preacher Bishop Fulton Sheen once observed that "millions of people hate the Church for what they think she teaches. But there aren't ten people who hate the Church for what she really teaches." This is never truer than when the topic of Catholic sexuality is raised. By now you've all seen the widely distributed press release from the office for the National Association of Conventional Wisdom on All Things Catholic

(NACWATC). For those of you who aren't in the loop, here's a copy of that famous document:

> **MEMO**
> **From: NACWATC**
> **To: The World**
>
> Please note. Roman Catholics think anything sexual is a sin and by the way, it's all Augustine's fault. Everyone knows that the Catholic Church is a backward, oppressive, patriarchal institution that tolerates sex only as a way of keeping its women barefoot and pregnant. Similarly, everyone knows – as Monty Python so helpfully pointed out – that as far as Catholics are concerned, every sperm is sacred and that the Church really doesn't want you to have sex unless a baby will definitely result every single time. And even then you should feel really, really guilty about it because enjoying yourself is absolutely, positively to be avoided by Catholics at all costs.
>
> At any rate, anything the Church teaches about sex – which is really very little anyway – is utter nonsense, so kindly ignore all those silly old men in their silly, pointy hats and go on about your business. Millions of people already ignore the Church on these issues. You should too. For fun and profit, please repeat this message as often as possible because, as we all know, saying something over and over automatically makes it true. Thank you. That is all.
>
> *NACWATC Steering Committee*

TWO FALSE IDEAS ATTRIBUTED TO THE CHURCH

Memos aside, I suspect the majority of people would be truly surprised to discover that most of what they think of as official Catholic teaching about sex has actually been officially denounced as a heresy by the Catholic Church at one point or another. This is especially true of the two predominant categories into which most people believe Catholic sexuality breaks down: *The Keep God Out of My Bedroom School* and *Aunt McGillicuddy's Antique Urn School.*

THE MEDITERRANEAN APPROACH

The Keep God Out of My Bedroom School of Sexuality has a very impressive alumni mailing list. Think of it as the more Mediterranean, *Must Leave Morning Mass Early So I Can Have Breakfast with My Mistress* school of thought. People who hold this view of sex tend to believe that "as long as I am a basically good person, occupy my mind with spiritual thoughts, let Father dip into my wallet whenever he asks, and don't miss Mass on Sundays and Holy Days, I can do whatever I want with my body, because, after all, God doesn't really care about what happens with those dangly bits as long as I shake them only at consenting adults behind closed doors."

Although many Catholics past and present do hold to this way of thinking about sex, there is nothing Catholic about it. In fact, it isn't remotely Christian — even in the broadest sense of the word. This school of thought has much more to do with a kind of low church gnosticism than it does with anything Christian.

Think of gnosticism as the RonCo knock-off of Christianity. It is to Christianity what GLH2000 — "spray-on hair-in-a-can" — is to real hair: a diverse group of religious movements that grew up alongside Christianity. Although looking like the name-brand product, they are cheap and shiny, making up in marketing what they lack in substance. This, of course, is exactly why people can't get enough of them even to this day. One of the common themes uniting the various gnostic movements is the idea that the body is largely irrelevant and even undesirable. According to the gnostics, man is primarily a spiritual being, inconveniently weighed down by a slab of meat (commonly referred to as "a body") that it is our great misfortune to lug about.

The less popular, high church gnostics dealt with this dim view of the body by punishing it with extreme fasting, strict abstinence, and harsh sexual continence. And sometimes castration and suicide.

These people weren't invited to a lot of parties.

By contrast, the people who threw the best parties, what I call the "low church gnostics," were a lot like our modern-day Keep God Out of My Bedroom Schoolers. They believed that since God only really cares about our spirits, we could do almost anything we wanted with our body, especially if it involved other people's bodies. After all, since our bodies are bad anyway, why not let them do the bad things they were made to do? Although there aren't a lot of high church gnostics around these days, the low church kind are in abundance. In the contemporary world, low church gnostics are the helpful folks who argue that the Catholic Church — and really, all Christendom — would be much better off if it would just stop obsessing about sex and be what God intended it to be: a glorified social service agency that stinks of incense and good intentions.

Despite its staying power, gnosticism in all its forms has been denounced as either outright paganism or a heresy since the second century A.D. by such prominent Christian writers as Melito of Sardis (died 190 A.D.), Irenaeus of Lyons (130–202 A.D.), and Tertullian (160–222 A.D.). In fact, in an intriguing discussion between Anglican archbishop of Canterbury Rowan Williams and John Paul II biographer George Weigel in 2007, low church gnosticism was fingered as Christianity's public enemy number one in the new millennium, for its ability both to seem Christian and to exhibit Christian piety all while undermining everything Christianity stands for as far as the body and relationship goes.

These prominent historical and contemporary Christians attacked gnosticism because, above all, Christianity is all about the body. The Christian knows that God doesn't love us just for our minds. He wants all of us. In fact, God loves us so much that he sent his Son to become one of us —

body and all! For the Christian, the scandal of the Incarnation is not that it reveals our bodies to be bad, but that it shows how incredibly good our bodies are and were always meant to be (see Gen. 1:31). As the Eastern Fathers of the Church put it, the incarnation divinized Human Nature (see CCC no. 460).

Therefore, gnosticism, especially the low church variety, fails in the light of Christianity because, for all its corporeal pessimism, it treats the body too *lightly*. To put it in colloquial terms, there's a reason nightclubs and singles bars are often called "meat markets" — even by the people who frequent them. Rather than thinking of the body as a creation of God deserving respect, latter-day gnostics treat their bodies as bags of meat, obsolete appendages — spiritual tonsils if you will — that have no bearing at all on their dignity as a human person or their eternal life. Therefore, the body can be treated with incredible irreverence and disregard — because, after all, it's worthless.

And yet, as the old saying goes, "God don't make junk." Catholic Christians know that matter (physical creation) *matters* to God. God took time out of the busiest schedule in the universe to make the body and pronounce it good (Genesis 1). Then, after the fall and by means of Christ's incarnation, passion, death, and resurrection, God went through a great deal of trouble to redeem us *and our bodies*. Salvation history is chock full of evidence that God is virtually obsessed with our bodiliness. In fact, both the Apostles' and the Nicene Creeds (if you don't profess 'em, you ain't Christian) emphasize the Christian belief in the resurrection of the body, meaning not only that our spirits will be raised to glory, but also that at the end of the world we will be reunited with our glorified bodies (just like Christ after the resurrection), spending our eternity as embodied beings (just like Christ now).

Considering how much time and attention God has given to the creation and redemption of our bodies, there should be no question that God cares a great deal about what we do with our bodies and how we treat others' bodies as well. The body is of quintessential importance because, as John Paul the Great said in his groundbreaking reflections on the theology of the body, "The body, in fact, and it alone is capable of making visible what is invisible — the spiritual and the divine. It was created to transfer into the visible reality of the world the mystery hidden since time immemorial in God and thus to be a sign of it."

Catholicism asserts that God cares about the body because his finger-prints are all over it. By prayerfully contemplating exactly how fearfully and wonderfully our physical bodies are made (Ps. 139:14), we can learn an immense amount about the nature of God himself, about God's plan for us and God's plan for harmonious and joyful human relationships. Understanding these things is essential to our happiness because if God is our maker and we are made in his image (Gen. 1:27), then our happiness depends upon our functioning according to our design. If you use a toaster in a manner that is inconsistent with its design, say, to pound nails, you don't end up with a happy toaster. In the same way, if we remain ignorant of the plan for a happy life and relationships that God encoded into the very fabric of our physical being, then we'll be doomed to function in a manner that leads to sickness, alienation, and misery rather than health, intimacy, and abundant joy.

Though God does care a great deal about our bodies and what we do with them, that does not mean that he doesn't want us to have fun with our bodies, or even enjoy the fullness of sexual pleasure. That's where the second heresy comes into play.

GETTING YER IRISH UP

Standing in contrast to the more Mediterranean, Keep God Out of My Bedroom School, Aunt McGillicuddy's Antique Urn School of Sexuality holds a more Anglo-Irish view. It grudgingly admits that sex is beauti-ful — in a grotesque, overdone, gothic sort of way — but above all, sex is *holy* and therefore, a little like Aunt McGillicuddy's antique urn, must be approached *delicately, cautiously,* and (ideally) *infrequently.* That is, "We oonly tooch it if we have to dust it, and then, only once a month er soo."

As far as the Church is concerned, the problem with this school of thought is twofold: it completely misconstrues the concept of holiness, and it overemphasizes the danger of sin hiding out behind every good thing. In the first instance, Aunt McGillicuddy-ites take Old Testament holiness and put a Jansenistic spin on it. Let me explain. In the Old Testament, holiness was something entirely "other" and "out there." God was *Elohim*, "God of the Mountain." He was so holy that you couldn't even say or write out his name. The holiest part of the Temple, the Holy of Holies, was so sacred that only the high priest could enter it, and then only once a year. In fact, this journey to the inner *sanctum sanctorum* was thought to be so dangerous that before the high priest could enter the Holy of Holies, his fellow priests would tie a rope around his waist so that if God decided to zap him while he was making his annual visit, his priestly colleagues could haul what was left of his toasted carcass out for something resembling a decent burial.

But in the New Testament, the Christian sense of holiness is radically different. In the person of Jesus Christ, true God became true Man. The "out there" became "right here." The utterly transcendent "I AM" became the immanent Emmanuel, "God with us." According to the *Catechism of the Catholic Church* (CCC), "the Word became flesh to be our model of holiness." Or, as St. Thomas Aquinas expresses it, "The only-begotten Son of God, wanting to make us sharers in his divinity, assumed our nature, so that he, made man, might make men gods" (CCC no. 460).

For the Catholic Christian, sex *is* holy, but not in the "touch it and die" sense of holiness. It is holy in the sense that it is the most complete and intimate way one divinized human person can give himself or herself to another divinized human person. Sex is holy because *you* are holy. God came to make it so. "You are a chosen race, a royal priesthood, a holy nation. . . . Once you were not a people, but now you are God's people!" (1 Pet. 2:9–10). In the words of Pope John Paul the Great, sex is a "self-gift." It is the sharing of all the holiness you are with all the holiness of another.

But if this was the only problem, then the McGillicuddy-ite's sense of holiness would simply be Judaic, not heretical. Where the Aunt McGillicuddy School really goes wrong is that it lumps a Jansenistic sense of sin on top of its Old Testament sense of holiness. In the early 1600s Cornelius Otto Jansen, a Scripture scholar and later Catholic bishop, asserted that human persons were so corrupted by original sin that we could not actually choose anything that was good. This teaching of the radical corruption of the human person essentially denied the saving power of baptism, which Catholics believe washes away original sin. Bishop Jansen wrote a controversial three-volume treatise on the theology of St. Augustine, which essentially distorted Augustine's teachings in the service of Jansen's radically morally corrupt view of the person (which, incidentally, is most likely the source of Augustine's oppressive sexual rep in today's conventional wisdom). Eventually, after a bitter dispute with the Holy See, Jansen's teachings became a heresy so un-Catholic it had to be denounced twice: it was formally condemned by Pope Urban VIII in 1643 and again by Pope Innocent X in 1653. In his famous work *Enthusiasm,* Msgr. Ronald Knox summarizes the Catholic problem with Jansenism by saying, "Jansenism never learned to smile. Its adherents forget, after all, to believe in grace, so hag-ridden are they by their sense of the need for it."

In other words, rightly recognizing that the potential for abuse exists when a person encounters any good thing, Jansenists assumed that people are utterly powerless to resist the temptation to abuse good things and therefore, all good things (and for the purposes of our discussion, especially sex) should be viewed with deep suspicion and avoided if possible.

Unfortunately, then, as now, people didn't just hop-to because the pope said so. Though the Church did what it could to institutionally rout out the scourge of Jansenism, the heresy had taken hold among the people and the clergy of France. In the 1600s Ireland was sending the vast majority of its seminarians to France for training. So Jansenism spread with a vengeance to Ireland and, following the mass emigration of Irish Catholics during the potato famine, it came to America, where it became easily accepted as the Official Catholic teaching on sex by our nation of apostate Puritans. (As a side note, many contemporary American Keep God Out of My Bedroom Schoolers are simply in reaction-formation to their Aunt McGillicuddy upbringing.)

Largely because of the lingering Jansenist impulses of nineteenth- and early twentieth-century Catholic America, Catholics and non-Catholics alike came to believe that "Catholics fear sex." But nothing could be further from the truth. Catholicism is the faith of celebration. It is the faith that *invented* holidays (literally, "Holy Days"). It is the faith about which the poet Hilaire Belloc famously wrote, "Wherever the Catholic sun doth shine / There is laughter, and music, and good red wine!" Catholicism is the faith that recognizes the holiness of all creation because of the miracle of Christ's incarnation. It is the faith of St. Francis of Assisi, who, when asked by his disciples whether to fast or feast when Christmas (the Feast of the Incarnation) fell on a Friday (traditionally a fast day) reportedly said, "It is my wish that on a day such as this even the walls should be smeared with meat so they may feast!" Only Catholic Christianity could hate a heresy because it "couldn't smile." And so while the world believes that Catholics hate and fear sex, the truth is even more scandalous. The truth is that the Catholic Church celebrates and esteems sex more than any other faith. By exploring what authentic Catholic tradition holds about human sexuality, any husband and wife can experience sex as God intended it to be experienced — an eye-popping, toe-curling, life-giving, profoundly sacred, and deeply spiritual union of one divinized human person with another.

REAL SEX EXPOSED

Just how much does Catholic tradition esteem sex? So much so that it incorporates sexual imagery into one of the core mysteries of the faith — the blessing of the baptismal font on the holiest night of the year, the Easter Vigil.

As a freshman in college, I was considering the priesthood, and I spent a year in the local diocesan seminary. My class was responsible for planning the Easter Vigil Mass that year, and we were going through the preparations with the seminary spiritual director. At the point where we were discussing the rites involved in the blessing of the baptismal font, our director, always on the lookout for a teachable moment, smiled and said, "Oh, that erotic rite."

Eleven pairs of eighteen-year-old eyebrows shot up.

He went on to explain that during the blessing of the font, the Easter candle was a phallic symbol plunged into the waters of the font to symbolize Christ impregnating the womb of the Church, from which new children of God would be born in the coming year. His words stunned me. Until that time, I'd believed what I had passively been taught by secular culture, that Catholicism, despite all its beauty, was essentially an erotophobic faith. And yet the Church had chosen to employ a powerful, symbolic, sexual act as the cornerstone of the chief sacrament of initiation, baptism. Since that time, I've discovered that various ancient rites of the Church have made even more graphic connections between human sexual love and the blessing of the font. For instance, in one rite, in addition to plunging the Easter candle into the font, the celebrant would also tip the candle so that melted wax would drip into the font, symbolically spilling the seed and completing the act that so beautifully signifies the fruitful marital union between Christ, the bridegroom, and the Church, his bride.

This will be shocking only to those who were raised to believe that Catholics fear and loathe sex. But despite what either Sr. Mary Attila or your sainted Ma and Da might have told you, of all the peoples who might hate their sexuality, authentic Catholics ain't among them.

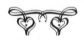

2 FOOL'S GOLD: HOLY SEX OR EROTICISM

The person is thus capable of a higher kind of love than [eroticism], which only sees objects as a means to satisfy one's appetites; the person is capable rather of friendship and self-giving, with the capacity to recognize and love persons for themselves. Like the love of God, this is a love capable of generosity. One desires the good of the other because he or she is recognized as worthy of being loved. This is a love which generates communion between persons, because each considers the good of the other as his or her own good. This is a self-giving made to one who loves us, a self-giving whose inherent goodness is discovered and activated in the communion of persons and where one learns the value of loving and of being loved.

— Pontifical Council for the Family
The Truth and Meaning of Human Sexuality

Most people confuse Holy Sex (which is really the only kind of sex worth having) with eroticism (which isn't really sex at all). During the American gold rush of the mid-1800s, amateur prospectors rushed to the West to make their fortunes. If they were lucky enough to survive the arduous journey, these countless victims bitten by the gold bug would spend hours and hours staking their claim, then digging, panning, and mining for that precious yellow metal.

Problem was, much of what the prospectors dug up and took to the assayer's office turned out to be pyrite, "fool's gold." Pyrite, an iron mineral, has a bronze-golden color and sparkles like the real McCoy, but it is virtually worthless.

The connection to sexuality is clear. Even in our allegedly sexually enlightened times, most people's sexual education, to the degree it happens at all, tends to focus simply on biology and mechanics. When it comes to romance and passion, people learn that from Hollywood, romance novels, daytime TV, their schoolmates, and porn. But these sources know nothing about Holy Sex. They only know about eroticism.

The only thing gold and iron pyrite have in common is that they are both shiny. The only thing that eroticism and Holy Sex have in common is that both are pleasurable — even extremely so. But that's where the similarities end.

HOLY SEX! DON'T SETTLE FOR SUBSTITUTES!

While the Bible lists eroticism as a sin (see Mark 7:21–22), Holy Sex is celebrated in the Song of Songs and in Ephesians as the sign of the union between Christ and the Church. To see how we're talking about two entirely different realities, let's do a side-by-side comparison between Holy Sex and eroticism:

Holy Sex	Eroticism
Very pleasurable	Very pleasurable
Driven by intimacy and arousal	Driven solely by arousal
Overcomes shame	Causes shame
Works for the good of the other	Uses the other
Welcomes children	Fears children
Shares the whole self	Withholds the self
More Joyful and vital with time	More Stagnant and boring with time (like a drug)
Gives life and health	Brings disease and death

Throughout this book, these differences will be highlighted in many ways, and of course some of these points overlap. For now, let's review some of these contrasting points to help orient ourselves to the profound differences between what people mistake for sex and the real article.

Very Pleasurable vs. Very Pleasurable

Both eroticism and Holy Sex are highly pleasurable, but even in this similarity, the beauty and pleasure of Holy Sex outstrips mere eroticism. This statement is either surprising or absurd to many people who either mistake eroticism for Holy Sex or, having had their sexual identities formed by eroticism, now live in negative reaction to it.

Think of eroticism as Las Vegas. Lots of neon, lots of flesh, lots of flash, and lots of noise. It can seem glamourous, dazzling, fascinating, and intoxicating. On the surface, there's a lot of fun to be had. You've probably heard the phrase "the glamour of evil" at one point or another. That's what we're talking about here. There's actually nothing wrong with glamour in itself, of course. But evil can use glamour as a shield to hide the slum in which it lives. Scratch the sexy surface, and the decay flows freely. Beneath the Vegas façade of flash, fun, and $4.99 prime rib is an empire with deep roots in criminality, the buying and selling of women, a tradition of taking advantage of the desperate poor and elderly, and an ethic of excess and degradation. In the same way, eroticism lures people in with promises of fun and fulfillment and dumps them out the back door dazed, depressed, and considerably worse off than when they started.

Worse, many people, having indulged too much in the "fun" of our Vegas-of-Eroticism, get burned or burned-out by the whole experience. They decide that it isn't just the *evil* that's evil, but also the glamour that evil often hides behind. As Pope Benedict XVI wrote in *Deus Caritas Est*, "The apparent exaltation of the body can quickly turn into a hatred of bodiliness." These people become entirely suspicious of sensuality. Rather than be tempted by the glamour of evil ever again, they remove glamour from their lives altogether. They renounce the bright lights and big city and hide out in an abandoned building where it's dark and quiet. Life becomes all work and no play. This is the puritanical sex of the Jansenists we discussed earlier: an empty, stripped-down, functional airplane hangar meant to be the corrective to the Vegas casino — but just as impoverished in its own way.

Most people believe that, when it comes to sex, there are only two choices: Vegas or the deserted building. Given that choice, only an idiot — or someone who has been deeply wounded — would choose to live in the airplane hangar. Human beings were created as *sensual* beings. That's why God gave us senses — to experience the world in all its glory as an invitation to know and love the Creator. If the only two choices held out to people are the light and sound phantasmagoria of the Vegas Strip or the bore-me-to-death functionality of the latest episode of *Style Me Puritan,* even considering the risks, most people will take their chances on the Strip. This is the problem faced by the Church. When it challenges eroticism, people mistakenly think that the only alternative is a stripped-down building. But nothing could be further from the truth.

The Church holds up Holy Sex as a third option — a positive alternative to the wretched, deadly excess of eroticism on one extreme and the puritanical pox on pleasure on the other. Compared to eroticism's Vegas, Holy Sex is every great cathedral and stained-glass window, every choir and orchestra, in one dynamic, God-given way of loving. Holy Sex is not glum sex, boring sex, polite sex, or joy-free sex. Neither is it exploitive sex, degrading sex, or loveless sex. Holy Sex is a passionate, sensual encounter between two lovers committed to a relationship that is faithful and forever — a relationship that has the power to raise up the couple in ecstasy toward the Divine, leading them beyond themselves and empowering them to touch the love of God himself.

Driven by Intimacy and Arousal vs. Driven Solely by Arousal

Think of arousal as the solid rocket boosters on the NASA space shuttle. They burn hot and fast but burn out quickly and are jettisoned once the shuttle has risen high into the atmosphere, after which the main fuel engine, intimacy, kicks in to take the astronauts to their destination.

Arousal is an important factor in the early stages of sexual intimacy for both Holy Sex and eroticism, but eroticism has nothing else to drive sex except arousal. Unfortunately, arousal, because it is a physiological state, is a very unreliable foundation for a long-term sexual relationship. If a couple relies only on arousal to stimulate their sexual relationship — as couples who practice eroticism do — then the sexual relationship will either stagnate over time as the pressures of life squeeze out the sense of chemistry that once existed between the couple, or the couple requires more and more "help" from outside sources such as porn in order to artificially create or inflate the arousal they are no longer capable of generating on a reliable basis.

By contrast, Holy Sex relies both on arousal and intimacy. Infallible Lovers are not opposed to taking advantage of the passionate spark that comes from chemistry and spontaneous arousal. They just don't leave their sexual relationship to the fates. Because of this, they work hard to maintain closeness all day long. Even on the days when they feel sick or stressed or tired, they still long for the comfort they find in the arms of their best friend, and even when they don't feel the immediate spark of arousal, the closeness generated by the warm feelings of friendship that increase as they lie in each other's arms often creates a longing to be even closer. This in turn kindles the fires of their sexual passion for one another. Where eroticism is all about drama, props, fireworks, and carnivals complete with dancing bears, Holy Sex is all about making each other always want just a little more until the glowing embers of passion burst into a surprising and sensual blaze.

Overcomes Shame vs. Causes Shame

Everyone wants to be loved totally and freely, but everyone is afraid that such a love will never find him or her. Most people are more used to being used — in ways large and small — than they are being loved.

In *Love and Responsibility*, Karol Wojtyla argued that shame, in the healthiest sense of the word, is a virtue that protects us from being used. Just as fear causes us to run from physical harm, and guilt causes us to run from moral harm, shame — in the healthiest sense of the word — is a feeling given to us by God that protects us from offenses against our dignity as human persons. Shame is the feeling that lets us know when other people are trying to use us as things rather than love us as people. In this sense, shame is actually a positive, protective emotion.

And yet, when we have been used by others to one extent or another, our sense of shame can become hyperactive — sort of like what happens if someone bumps into your old football or dancing injury. The exacerbated sense of shame that comes from being treated like an object can alienate us from others and even keep us from God. In the book of Genesis, shame was experienced only after the Fall, when Adam and Eve first realized they were naked, "and they were ashamed." Adam and Eve, of course, were naked before the Fall as well, but it wasn't a problem. Before the regrettable apple incident, Adam and Eve didn't see their nakedness as a liability. They experienced it as freedom, as a sign of their dignity as persons and the safety they experienced in the union they enjoyed with God and each other. It was only after the Fall that Adam and Eve came to realize that they had another option besides loving and respecting each other. Now, they discovered, they could use each other as well. Original sin ruptured the protection Adam and Eve enjoyed as a result of their original union with God and each other. For the first time, humans felt that their nakedness, rather than being a witness to the joy and holy vulnerability they experienced in the presence of God and each other, was a sign that they were alone, alienated, exposed, and capable of using and being used by one another. With this realization came a sense of shame, which was intended as an early warning system designed to protect each person from using or being used.

People today still experience this shame when others seek to use them in one way or another. But Holy Sex — lovemaking that occurs in the free union of a married man and woman — allows a couple to safely overcome the overactive sense of shame that causes people to hold back when they ought to give themselves more freely to each other and to God. When a husband and wife in a truly committed, loving, generous, and respectful relationship make love with one another, they are given the grace, over time, to overcome their temptation to use one another or fear being used by one another. As a result, they can begin to get a tiny taste of the unity our first parents enjoyed with God and each other before the Fall. Man can never return to Eden. That paradise is lost to us until the next life. But through the grace of matrimony, man and woman can set up house in a neighborhood near Eden, and they can breathe in the fragrance of that garden wafting through their windows, giving them joy in the present and hinting at great things to come.

By contrast, eroticism, because it is all about using people as if they were toys, *increases* our sense of shame. Remember, shame is the feeling that warns us we're being treated as things rather than being loved as people. When you allow yourself to use others, or permit yourself to be used by others, shame grows. At first, that shame causes us to be distrustful of others. "I thought he loved me. I'm never going to let anyone hurt me like that again." (For more information, see chapter 8, especially the discussion of "defensive attachment," pp. 134ff.) Even when others approach you in love, you'll tend to wonder what they *really* want from you. You'll be more likely to put up barriers to their love and make others prove themselves to you before you will give your heart again — if ever.

If you continue to allow yourself to be used by eroticism, you'll become alienated, not just from others, but also from yourself. You'll become so convinced that your only worth is derived from being the object of others' desire that you stop noticing or minding you're being used. You'll come to make a circus act out of your sexuality, publicly claiming "liberation" while privately struggling with self-hatred and the eating disorders, cutting, drinking, drugs, and other excesses people use to numb their psychic and spiritual pain.

Works for the Good of the Other vs. Uses the Other

As you can see in our discussion of shame, eroticism is primarily concerned with what it can get out of the other person without having to give too much in return.

You can see this most dramatically with regard to casual sex, where people get to know each other as little as they need to in order to get each other's goodies, but it applies in more subtle forms to marriage as well. Wives, in particular, complain to me all the time about otherwise loving men who pout and become angry if their wives ask to take the night off from love-making. And husbands complain to me about wives who never want to be intimate until their wives are trying to "soften them up" to get something else out of them. Both are examples of how we treat sex as a right and our lover as a vending machine designed for our gratification rather than a person deserving of love and respect.

In either case, when this happens, sex ceases to really be about love and becomes a means to an end — the lover, merely a tool that you use to help you achieve your goal. After a while, this dynamic leads to the shame we discussed above and causes sexual intimacy in marriage to die.

Holy Sex, by comparison, always seeks the good of the other person. Infallible Lovers recognize that even though sex is perhaps the most intimate way for a couple to celebrate their love for one another, it isn't the only way. While the lover schooled in eroticism always feels compelled to use sex as "the best and only way I can really show anyone I care or allow myself to feel cared for," the Infallible Lover is totally free to choose the best way to be loving to the beloved *in this moment*. Sometimes that will mean doing something other than having sex — things like watching the baby, or cleaning up the house, or just talking, praying, or cuddling. And when the couple practicing Holy Sex decides to celebrate the fullness of their friendship by making love, they make sure they don't treat each other in a way that turns the other person into a thing.

Infallible Lovers never restrain their passion for one another, but they are always mindful that *love* is the point of lovemaking, not creating some sexual drama. It can require some negotiation to work out the boundaries of what is appropriate and what is not (we'll discuss this in a later chapter). But those who have been misled to believe that the Church is "down on sex" will be surprised to learn that aside from a very few specific requirements, very little is actually forbidden to lovers celebrating Holy Sex. Playfulness and passion, erotic language, virtually every sexual position, or the use of attractive clothing and lingerie or other means of heightening the sensuality of lovemaking can be perfectly acceptable parts of Infallible Loving. That said, *creating new experiences is never the primary point of Holy Sex.* Celebrating the couple's love for one another is. Infallible Lovers always make sure to discuss how to keep their sexual relationship fresh and exciting while still respecting the fact that sex is primarily about loving each other, not about creating an ever-expanding repertoire of feats of sexual derring-do.

Welcomes Children vs. Fears Children

Because eroticism is "all about me" and how much I can get out of you without having to give too much in return (e.g., commitment, fidelity, or real love), it is terrified of children. Because eroticism itself is childish, it sees children as competition for limited resources that the adult child would put to "better" use indulging himself or herself. Furthermore, like bacteria exposed to the sunlight, eroticism tends to die in the presence of real love. What happens when a child comes along? If your sex lives are rooted in eroticism, you tend to see your sexual relationship take a nose-dive. This is because eroticism tells you that sex is entirely about recreation. As soon as something more meaningful than mere recreation comes along — like loving and nurturing children — sex become just one more formerly fun thing you don't have the time or energy for.

Holy Sex, by contrast, because it always considers what's good for the other person first and is rooted in a real love, welcomes children. Infallible Lovers bow to the mystery through which authentic love becomes another living, breathing person. Further, when children arrive on the scene, Infallible Lovers, who have been practicing generous love all along, are able to also find the generosity required to keep their love and passion alive. Because their relationship — especially their sexual relationship — is fueled by generosity, Infallible Lovers recognize that anything that challenges them to be more generous actually makes them better lovers, so even though they are aware of the work involved in parenting, they recognize childrearing as a labor of love that leads to even greater loving.

We'll examine this in greater depth in chapter 9 on the Fifth Power of Holy Sex: the power to create.

Shares the Whole Self vs. Withholds the Self

Eroticism only gives as much of myself as I *must* give to get what I want. Outside of marriage, sexual partners will often withhold their hearts from one another, choosing only to give or take whatever pleasure their bodies can generate. This is sad, because it is so impoverished. As we've observed, there is nothing wrong with pleasure. Eroticism is not a sin because it is pleasurable. It is sinful because it involves giving less than the lovers deserve to receive from one another. When a couple has Holy Sex, they are speaking a language that transcends words and says, "Everything I am, I now give to you." But eroticism causes our bodies to make certain promises that our minds, hearts, and spirits don't intend to keep. The problem is that healthy human beings really don't know how to check their hearts, minds, and spirits at the door. Of course, we can engage in eroticism so much that it causes our bodies, minds, hearts, and souls to become dis-integrated, in which case, we don't even know how wounded we are. Suffice it to say that if you're the type of person who knows how to check your heart, mind, or spirit at the door, then you'll have a lot of work to do before you can become an Infallible Lover, because despite your best intentions, over time, anyone you love will be left wondering if your lovemaking is less about love and more about scratching a sexual itch.

Even in marriage, couples can hold back from each other. For instance, I'm often shocked by couples who think that praying together is "too intimate." What do they think sex is? Unless they learn to share their souls, such a couple will never be able to experience Holy Sex, because Holy Sex is a kind of prayer. If you don't challenge yourselves to share your souls outside the bedroom, you won't be able to share your souls *in* the bedroom, and your lovemaking will suffer because less than all of you will be showing up for the experience.

Another way couples withhold from each other is through contraception. We'll discuss this more in chapter 9 on the Fifth Power of Holy Sex, as well as in chapter 10 on Natural Family Planning, but for now, it is important to know that any time a husband and wife contracept, they are saying to each other, "I just want the parts of you that make me feel good; I don't want the parts of you that make me commit to you for life and enable us to celebrate a love so powerful it could become its own life." That doesn't mean that a couple must intend to have a baby every time they have sex. But it means that Infallible Lovers are mindful that pregnancy is not a sexually transmitted disease to be avoided at all costs. Rather, Infallible Lovers know that life is the logical fruit of a faithful and lifelong sexual relationship. The couple, to be truly Infallible Lovers to one another, must be mature enough to not fear the life-giving power of their love. After all, as Scripture tells us, "Perfect love casts out fear" (1 John 4:18). Holy Sex is a celebration of our striving for that perfect love between man and woman made possible by God's grace. "Be not afraid!"

Infallible Lovers don't hold back from one another — they *can't.* God tells us that he is a "jealous God" (Exod. 20:5). Our Divine Lover wants all of us. He doesn't want just the parts we care to give him. He wants us to love him with everything, and he wants to love us with everything he has to give us in return. In the same way, Holy Sex — as a physical sign of God's own love for the lovers — demands that the lovers hold nothing back. Holy Sex wants to set the bodies, minds, hearts, and souls of the lovers on fire. Holy Sex wants to stamp God's own love on every part of the lovers. Holy Sex, unlike eroticism, never says, "Just give me your various body parts, thanks." Rather, it says, "Give me everything! I want it all. I want to burn my name into your body, mind, heart, and soul and yours in mine. I want to love you so passionately that I can see my unborn children in your eyes." When you can say all those things to your beloved, you are an Infallible Lover.

More Joyful and Vital with Time
vs. More Stagnant and Boring with Time (like a Drug)

Eroticism, as we've seen, does not make love the primary point of lovemaking. It sees sex as an experience and the point of lovemaking creating new exciting experiences. Love really isn't a major concern of the person or couple with eroticism on their minds. Love may be there, or it may not, but as long as the sexual experience achieves some degree of sensual release, then the couple with an eroticized mind-set considers sex to be good.

It bears repeating: the problem with this mind-set isn't that it values sexual pleasure. Pleasure is good. But sex without love — or with diminished love — is like a drug that requires higher and higher doses to allow the addict to achieve the same high. Sex without love requires the couple to seek out more and more dramatic experiences to get the same high each time — the high that love would otherwise supply. There are two possible results. Either the couple eventually hits a line that one or the other will not cross and as a result, passion dies and frustration reigns, or the couple keeps pushing the limits of sexual experience until the boundaries that protect the dignity and integrity of the marital relationship completely collapse, and the marriage falls apart.

Holy Sex, however, is always fresh and exciting. Of course, Infallible Lovers value passion and sensuality and are open to trying new things that allow them to be more vulnerable and joyful with one another. But because they make *love* the point of lovemaking, their love for one another makes sex rewarding and intimate, even when they're unable to pull out all the stops. The love, partnership, friendship, respect, and caring they share all day with one another is the substance of their lovemaking, and sensual experience is the sweet icing on the cake. Where eroticism is happy only with the most sickeningly sweet desserts, Infallible Lovers know that while some cakes have more icing than others, anything they bake together will be delicious. And their culinary skills only get better. Because Infallible Lovers root their lovemaking in intimacy seasoned with sensuality, Holy Sex becomes more passionate with time. Even when a couple is sick or stressed and unable to muster the energy for a fireworks display, they still long to have their best friend's arms wrapped around them. And they can use these quieter times of lovemaking to refresh and communicate their desire and commitment to create some more dramatic fireworks at some point in the future.

Gives Life and Health vs. Brings Disease and Death

The last contrast we'll examine is the tendency of eroticism to cause sickness and death versus the power of Holy Sex to create health and life.

Romans 6:23 tells us that the "wages of sin are death." That's a hard saying, but it happens to be true. People everywhere think that sin and pleasure are synonymous, and that was certainly true for the Puritans but it's never been true for Catholics. Again, eroticism is sinful not because it is pleasurable, but because it treats people as things and it causes people to use their bodies, minds, hearts, and souls in a way they were never designed to be used. If you use a curling iron to stir your spaghetti sauce, or your MP3 player to spread peanut butter and jelly on your bread, or your DVDs to play Frisbee with your dog, these things will break because they were not designed to be used this way. Likewise, the human body, mind, heart, and soul were not designed for eroticism, and when they are used for eroticism, they break down.

St. Thomas Aquinas told us that "grace builds on nature." In other words, grace-filled moments make us stronger, healthier, better functioning people. By contrast, sin tears nature apart. It causes us to do things with our bodies, minds, and spirits that they were not designed to do until our bodies, minds, and souls fall apart. Eroticism is not sinful because it is pleasurable. It is sinful because it destroys.

How does it destroy? Psychologically, emotionally, and physically. Here's one example. As shown in research published in the journal *Pediatrics*, young adults who are promiscuous have higher rates of depression and emotional problems. Interestingly, research clearly shows that it is not that depressed people are having more promiscuous sex to make themselves feel better, but rather it is promiscuous sex that is causing depression. By contrast, studies show that couples engaged in what I call Holy Sex are actually happier and mentally healthier because of their sexual relationship. Holy Sex is grace-filled; therefore it builds on nature. Eroticism is sinful; therefore it tears nature apart.

Eroticism causes physical problems as well. According to the Centers for Disease Control, there are 19 million new STD infections in the United States each year, costing an already strained healthcare system 14.1 billion dollars annually. Sexually transmitted diseases like gonorrhea, syphilis, herpes, and AIDS, to name a few, are communicated by eroticism, but they are not transmitted by Holy Sex because it is always faithful and respectful of the natural order. A couple engaged in Holy Sex is at zero risk for these and other diseases (except in cases where one of them has contracted a disease prior to their marriage). But eroticism causes sickness and death. Why? Because the body, mind, heart, and soul were not designed for eroticism.

More than preventing illness and death, Holy Sex actually makes people healthier and enables them to live longer. One 2007 study published in the *Journal of Epidemiology and Community Health* found that unmarried people were 58 percent more likely to die over the eight-year study than marrieds. In general, research on marriage and health outcomes consistently shows that couples who are in healthy, faithful marriages live longer than others, are more mentally healthy than others, and are at lower risk for many physical diseases — not just STDs.

WHEN LOVE GOES BAD

These various side-by-side comparisons reveal the challenge for those who are in-the-know about Holy Sex. When the Church talks about sex and says that it's beautiful, life-giving, self-donative (i.e., self-giving), generous, and "so precious that it deserves to be saved for marriage where it can be a path of purification, holiness, and wholeness," the Church is talking only about Holy Sex. But when people — marinated as they are in a culture of eroticism — hear what the Church is saying about sex, they mistakenly think the Church is talking about eroticism. This is why they scoff.

Imagine a bunch of would-be prospectors who all got burned by an iron-pyrite scam. They meet a prospector running into town screaming, "I've found gold! Look! Real gold! I'll share it with all of you! We're rich! Don't you see? We're rich!" Do the sad-sack fool's gold prospectors rejoice at the generosity of this newest miner on the scene? Of course not. They assume the newbie to be as stupid as they were. They dismiss him and insult him. At best they humor him. And in every case, they think him an idiot for making so much out of nothing. In the same way, when the Church preaches the beauty and power of Holy Sex to a world wounded and objectified by eroticism, people have two reactions. They dismiss the Church's teaching as the idealized, demented mutterings of a bunch of old men with funny religious garb who don't have the first idea what they're talking about. Or they are scandalized and offended that the Church would make so much out of so little. Some especially talented NACWATC-funded pundits do a little of both. And that's just the way Satan wants it.

Think of eroticism as Satan's plagiarism of Holy Sex, the most powerful force in the world, the only force that can physically, psychologically, and spiritually weld people into one and create life welcomed by the lovers. Satan can't let something like that go unchallenged. So what does he do? He must plagiarize it. He must destroy it.

Many of you might be rolling your eyes right now. After all, Satan doesn't *really* exist right? We don't believe that nonsense anymore, do we? Well, I do, and I'm confident you would, too, if you looked into the eyes of a child who had been serially raped by his uncles, or the walking-dead expression on a hooker's face, or even the face of a woman whose playfulness and vitality have been robbed by too many demeaning "relationships." Evil can be so palpable and insidiously creative that it deserves its own name. Christians name the source of that evil Satan.

Eroticism represents some of Satan's best work. Satan's plan for destroying Holy Sex is to soak us in eroticism and spoil us by it so that we never even consider what Holy Sex is really all about. Each and every one of us has been affected and influenced by eroticism, and this makes it harder to understand what the Church really means when it talks about Holy Sex.

While eroticism inevitably spells the death of both the person and the culture-at-large, Holy Sex is the hope for health and life for generations to come. The reason the Church makes such a big deal out of sex is because sex is the building block of civilization. None of us would be here if it wasn't for sex. Culture and civilizations would not exist without people. People would not exist if not for sex. If Satan can alter our views about the nature of sex, if he can divorce sex from our physicality and make it all about feelings, then he can alter our views about what constitutes a healthy person, a healthy family, and he can ultimately distort our capacity to have a healthy, vibrant culture. A culture whose major export is a multibillion dollar porn industry is a culture that has lost its capacity to experience the fullness of beauty, truth, goodness, and humanity. But a culture that celebrates Holy Sex recognizes that humankind, while coming from the animals, is higher than the animals and set apart for greater things. A culture that celebrates Holy Sex is a culture that knows what it takes to be a healthy person; it is a culture that protects and values healthy, intact families in which children can experience all the benefits of having both a mother and a father living under the same roof with them. It is a culture in which these children — who are neither a surprise nor unwanted because people are not shocked by the fact that sex actually results in babies — grow to achieve their full potential to become healthy citizens of both the world and the Kingdom of God, capable of exhibiting the heights of human capacity for beauty, goodness, and truth, and capable of experiencing a sensuality that raises the whole world "in ecstasy toward the Divine."

I think that's a battle worth fighting. Don't you? All I can say to the neo-gnostic, NACWATC crowd is that if the Catholic Church is the only institution remaining after nearly 1,930 years of universal agreement among Christians of every denomination on this topic with the courage to fight that battle, then so be it. As historians like Thomas Woods and Thomas Cahill have observed, the Catholic Church has been charged with saving civilization before. She can do it again.

Only this time, maybe she can do it with you and your beloved, since now you too know the truth.

3 WHAT ARE INFALLIBLE LOVERS MADE OF?

Become what you are.
— Pope John Paul II, *Familiaris Consortio*

"Chastity is a virtue. . . .
Whoever prays for it will certainly attain it."
— St. Alphonsus Ligouri

Catholic sexuality is a profound and joyful thing. It is superior to what any other philosophy of sex has to offer because it insists that we respect the gift of our own humanity, as well as the humanity of our lover, and it compels us to appreciate the power we invoke when we share ourselves with that one person God has chosen for us. Furthermore, Catholic sexuality is really about the communication of one whole person with another — with all that means. To be an Infallible Lover means to be committed to becoming a healthy, faithful person who knows how to communicate the fullness of his or her being to another healthy, faithful person. Who wouldn't want to celebrate a sexuality based on such a reality?

In this next step of our exploration into what Holy Sex is (and what it isn't), we need to look at the ingredients that go into a healthy sexuality. It isn't unusual for me to get calls from prospective clients who want only to talk about problems in their sexual relationship. Only reluctantly will they allow me to review the relationship as a whole. They feel like I'm looking for trouble. I'm not, of course. The problem is that Holy Sex is not some artificial appendage that can be taken out of the drawer and strapped onto the person when it's needed. Holy Sex is an expression of the whole person. As the Pontifical Council for the Family explains in its very helpful and accessible document *The Truth and Meaning of Human Sexuality*, sex "concerns the intimate nucleus of the person."

You really can't think about sex — and you certainly can't do effective sex therapy — unless you place it in the context of the overall health of the relationship. Many secular sex therapists would take issue with this statement. They believe that sex therapy is just about finding the right amount of friction and lubrication to get the job — defined as biological satisfaction — done. While that may be enough for eroticism, that doesn't even begin to approach Holy Sex. Frankly, it isn't even enough for eroticism, which is never satisfied with just getting Part A to fit snugly into Part B. Eroticism wants passion. It wants spirit. It wants to be vital and whole and beautiful. It wants to live! But because it's just a dim shadow of the real thing, it can never be anything more than what it is — a biological urge that becomes a means of self-medication for suffering people who don't yet have what it takes to make real intimacy happen.

So what does it take to be an Infallible Lover? It takes a commitment to be a whole and healthy person. That doesn't mean you have to have achieved total health and wholeness, just that you need to be striving for it and willing to see your sexual relationship, not just as a thing you do, but mainly as an expression of who you are. Further, it means that if you are struggling sexually, the root of the problem most likely has more to do with your character or relationship than it does with mechanics and proper lighting. Your sexual relationship is a microcosm of everything good and bad in your entire relationship.

In my book for parents, *Beyond the Birds and the Bees,* I describe eight virtues that stand at the heart of Holy Sex. Infallible Lovers strive not only to master the techniques that enhance sexual pleasure but also to master the virtues that make it possible for them to be healthy people and enviable partners who are capable of celebrating an eye-popping, toe-curling, deeply spiritual, and profoundly soulful sexuality.

HOW TO BECOME AN INFALLIBLE LOVER:
A RECIPE

We have all heard the nursery rhyme that tells us that girls are made of "sugar and spice and everything nice" and that boys are made of "snakes and snails and puppy dog tails." Be that as it may, here's the recipe real men and real women follow to learn how to become Infallible Lovers to one another.

> 1 cup Love (for best results, use self-donative variety)
>
> 1 cup Responsibility (mix ½ cup self-discipline with ½ cup stewardship)
>
> 1 cup Faith
>
> 1 cup Respect (combine ½ cup self-respect and ½ cup respect for others)
>
> 1 cup Intimacy (combine equal parts verbal and emotional communication)
>
> 1 cup Cooperation
>
> 1 cup Joy
>
> 1 cup Personhood (combine a sense of being made in the image of God with a heaping tablespoon of — choose one of the following — masculinity or femininity)

Bake slowly over a lifetime.

WHAT ABOUT CHASTITY?

As you look at that recipe, some of you might be wondering why I haven't included chastity in the mix. The reason chastity is not *in* the mix is that chastity *is* the mix. Many people are under the mistaken impression that chastity is the same thing as repression. (All those jokes about "chastity belts" haven't helped matters in this regard.) But chastity is really the ability to apply in the sexual sphere all of the virtues I mention above.

Chastity is what enables me to be truly free to make a gift of myself at the right time, in the right way, with the right person. Chastity isn't just for people who aren't married. It's for everyone, because everyone needs to know the best time, place, and manner by which they can be most loving to the person they love. I can say that I am chaste, not if I simply keep my genitals locked up, but rather if I know how to be loving, responsible, respectful, intimate, cooperative, joyful, faithful, and fully human in re-lationship to my sexuality. Keeping one's genitals under lock and key — literally or metaphorically — is not chastity. It is repression. And not even the allegedly "uber-repressive, sexually backward, head-in-the-sand, sour-faced, grimly pious Catholic Church" defines chastity as repression. In fact, the *Catechism of the Catholic Church* says, "Chastity means the successful integration of sexuality within the person and thus the inner unity of man in his bodily and spiritual being" (CCC no. 2337). Or, to put it another way, here is what the *Encyclopedia of Catholic Doctrine* has to say on the matter.

> Chastity is the virtue that enables one to use one's sexual powers properly. The chaste person is in control of his or her sexual desires rather than being controlled by them. Necessary for both the married and the unmarried, chastity is rooted in a deep respect for the other person, who should never be used merely as an object to satisfy one's sexual desires.... Chastity allows one to avoid viewing others, even one's spouse, as a sexual object and to have the love and friendship for others, especially one's spouse, that one ought to have.

Clearly, contrary to what both conventional wisdom and the dues-paying members of NACWATC would have you believe, there is more to chastity than white-knuckling it until one says "I do," after which, "anything goes."

Where *do* people get this stuff, anyway?

To say that Infallible Lovers are chaste, then, means that at all times they strive to be fully loving to their spouse in a way that is desirable, appropriate to the situation, and considerate of the best interests of their mate. There is a saying that "when all you've got is a hammer, every problem looks like a nail." Fallible lovers, because they are unchaste in their marriages, tend to have only a hammer. They know that sex is the most intimate way to express love to their mate, so they think it's the only way to express love to their mate — or at least, the only way that really matters. Fallible lovers will put up with conversation, cuddling, compliments, physical affection, and "sweet nothings" only to the degree that they lead to sex. And on those occasions when these things don't end up with fireworks in the bedroom, fallible lovers become pouting, resentful, withdrawn, and irritable.

Infallible Lovers, because they are chaste, love to make love, but they also know that there is more to lovemaking than sex. They work hard to be as fully loving as they are able — and as circumstances permit — all day long. Infallible Lovers may still *want* to ravish each other in the produce aisle of the grocery store, or when the little ones are underfoot, or when one's mate has the flu, but they recognize that — in these situations at least — offering to go to the other side of the store to get the forgotten milk, offering to watch the kids while one's mate takes some time to relax, or suddenly appearing with a hot cup of tea and box of fluffy tissues are perhaps even more beautiful expressions of love than sex. In other words, the virtues that make up chastity enable Infallible Lovers to avoid becoming resentful when the urge to make love can't be immediately expressed. They look for the fullest way they can make a gift of themselves to their mate in the moment. This leads to truly remarkable lovemaking when the moment finally arrives for their bodies to speak that language that goes beyond words and says, "Look what perfect partners we are! Everything we are works for each other's good. Even our bodies were made for each other!"

That is what authentic chastity looks like in action — as the Church *really* defines it. Infallible Lovers cultivate the eight virtues that lie at the heart of Holy Sex so that they can be truly chaste lovers — lovers who are fully loving all the time, not just when one of them experiences an itch that needs to be scratched.

In the following pages, we'll examine each of the eight virtues that empower you to become an Infallible Lover. First, take a moment to evaluate how well you express each of the virtues both in your everyday life and in your sexual relationship with your partner. The following quiz can help you identify your strengths as well as those areas that may require some shoring up.

Quiz
BAKER'S QUIZ

The following questions address each of the identified ingredients of Infallible Loving in general, not simply in the sexual area of your life. Think about your relationship as a whole when you answer them, not just your sexual relationship with your mate. Incidentally, the following quiz is not intended to be a comprehensive diagnostic measure of your true capacity for each of the eight virtues. Better to think of it as a kind of examination of conscience to evaluate your potential as an Infallible Lover.

Directions

Write your score for each section of the quiz and then tally up all the scores to discover the degree to which you exhibit the ingredients of Infallible Loving. Once you've completed the quiz, pay attention to which areas are strengths and which areas need improvement. The remainder of the chapter will suggest some ways you can develop other virtues in your life and relationship. Discuss these opportunities for improvement with your spouse, and see if the two of you can come up with additional ways to encourage each other to become Infallible Lovers. If you and your mate are reading the book together (which I recommend) both of you should take the quiz separately and discuss why you answered as you did.

1. Self-Donative Love

1. I am mindful of the goals and values that are important to my partner, and every day I work, in concrete ways, to help him or her pursue those goals and values.

Disagree Totally	Disagree Somewhat	Neither Agree nor Disagree	Agree Somewhat	Agree Totally
1	2	3	4	5

2. I willingly and cheerfully take on the challenges, responsibilities, and sacrifices of marriage and family life.

Disagree Totally	Disagree Somewhat	Neither Agree nor Disagree	Agree Somewhat	Agree Totally
1	2	3	4	5

3. My mate would agree that I am an attentive, sensitive, generous, and thoughtful spouse.

Disagree Totally	Disagree Somewhat	Neither Agree nor Disagree	Agree Somewhat	Agree Totally
1	2	3	4	5

4. My spouse and family get the best of me (as opposed to what's left of me after I am done with my work, friends, community involvements, and hobbies).

Disagree Totally	Disagree Somewhat	Neither Agree nor Disagree	Agree Somewhat	Agree Totally
1	2	3	4	5

5. I willingly and generously respond to my mate's requests and needs, even the ones that challenge my comfort zone (assuming they don't violate my moral standards).

Disagree Totally	Disagree Somewhat	Neither Agree nor Disagree	Agree Somewhat	Agree Totally
1	2	3	4	5

6. I do not belittle or criticize the things or interests that my spouse enjoys but I myself do not appreciate. Instead, I work to find the truth, goodness, and beauty in all the things my mate finds true, good, and beautiful.

Disagree Totally	Disagree Somewhat	Neither Agree nor Disagree	Agree Somewhat	Agree Totally
1	2	3	4	5

Self-Donative Love score: _____ *out of a possible 30 points.*

2. Responsibility

(½ cup self-discipline; ½ cup stewardship)

1. I am good at delaying gratification in any area of my life. If circumstances require me to wait or "do without" for a time, I can be happy and content while I wait.

Disagree Totally	Disagree Somewhat	Neither Agree nor Disagree	Agree Somewhat	Agree Totally
1	2	3	(4)	5

2. I am attentive and responsive to the needs of my spouse and family, even when I feel like doing something else.

Disagree Totally	Disagree Somewhat	Neither Agree nor Disagree	Agree Somewhat	Agree Totally
1	(2)	3	4	5

3. The people in my life know that they are more important than the things I have. For instance, I clean, maintain, and care for the things God has given me, but not to the degree that people are afraid to use the things God has given me. (e.g., "Welcome to my home / look at my car — but don't touch anything!")

Disagree Totally	Disagree Somewhat	Neither Agree nor Disagree	Agree Somewhat	Agree Totally
1	*2*	3	4	5

4. I am good at both expressing my emotions and controlling them, and I know the appropriate times to do either.

Disagree Totally	Disagree Somewhat	Neither Agree nor Disagree	Agree Somewhat	Agree Totally
1	*2*	3	4	5

5. I am good at keeping my priorities in order. (I do not feel pulled in a million different directions all of the time.)

Disagree Totally	Disagree Somewhat	Neither Agree nor Disagree	Agree Somewhat	Agree Totally
1	2	3	4	5

6. I am good at balancing meeting my own needs with meeting the needs of others.

Disagree Totally	Disagree Somewhat	Neither Agree nor Disagree	Agree Somewhat	Agree Totally
1	*2*	3	4	5

Responsibility score: __13__ *out of a possible 30 points.*

3. Faith

1. I am attentive to the spiritual dimensions of everyday life.

Disagree Totally 1	Disagree Somewhat 2	Neither Agree nor Disagree 3	Agree Somewhat ④	Agree Totally 5

2. I have an active prayer life that consists of formal and casual prayer, as well as regular participation in the sacraments, and I am comfortable praying with my spouse.

Disagree Totally 1	Disagree Somewhat 2	Neither Agree nor Disagree ③	Agree Somewhat 4	Agree Totally 5

3. I am able to discern God speaking to me through the events of my everyday life.

Disagree Totally 1	Disagree Somewhat 2	Neither Agree nor Disagree 3	Agree Somewhat ④	Agree Totally 5

4. I seek to live my life according to Scripture and the teachings of the Church, and I constantly strive to develop a deeper understanding and appreciation of both.

Disagree Totally 1	Disagree Somewhat 2	Neither Agree nor Disagree 3	Agree Somewhat ④	Agree Totally 5

5. I have a faith that is both emotionally fulfilling and intellectually well-informed.

Disagree Totally 1	Disagree Somewhat 2	Neither Agree nor Disagree 3	Agree Somewhat ④	Agree Totally 5

6. I am capable of explaining and defending important moral and spiritual teachings of the Church in rational, meaningful ways.

Disagree Totally	Disagree Somewhat	Neither Agree nor Disagree	Agree Somewhat	Agree Totally
1	2	3	④	5

Faith score: **23** out of a possible 30 points.

4. Respect

(½ cup self-respect; ½ cup respect for others)

1. I am capable of making other people take me seriously.

Disagree Totally	Disagree Somewhat	Neither Agree nor Disagree	Agree Somewhat	Agree Totally
1	2	③	4	5

2. I do not do things that will demean my God-given personal dignity or threaten my moral well-being, even if someone I care about becomes irritated with me for taking that position.

Disagree Totally	Disagree Somewhat	Neither Agree nor Disagree	Agree Somewhat	Agree Totally
1	②	3	4	5

3. I do not refuse the requests of others lightly. I do not refuse people simply because I don't feel like doing what they have asked. I respond to all requests that I believe are reasonable, and I at least give a fair hearing to those requests that are suspect to me before deciding how to respond.

Disagree Totally	Disagree Somewhat	Neither Agree nor Disagree	Agree Somewhat	Agree Totally
1	2	3	④	5

4. I expect each member of my family to do as much as they can to take care of our home and each other. I am good at making this happen.

Disagree Totally	Disagree Somewhat	Neither Agree nor Disagree	Agree Somewhat	Agree Totally
1	2	3	(4)	5

5. I know how to dress in a way that is attractive, but not intentionally provocative.

Disagree Totally	Disagree Somewhat	Neither Agree nor Disagree	Agree Somewhat	Agree Totally
1	(2)	3	4	5

6. I make sure to tell the people I love how special and important they are to me every day, and I show that specialness in my behavior toward them.

Disagree Totally	Disagree Somewhat	Neither Agree nor Disagree	Agree Somewhat	Agree Totally
1	(2)	3	4	5

Respect score: __17__ *out of a possible 30 points.*

5. Intimacy

(combine equal parts verbal and emotional communication)

1. I am good at *respectfully* expressing my feelings.

Disagree Totally	Disagree Somewhat	Neither Agree nor Disagree	Agree Somewhat	Agree Totally
1	(2)	3	4	5

2. My spouse would say that I am a good and thoughtful listener.

Disagree Totally	Disagree Somewhat	Neither Agree nor Disagree	Agree Somewhat	Agree Totally
1	②2	3	4	5

3. I regularly ask my spouse to discuss things that are important to him or her, even if they don't interest me in the same way.

Disagree Totally	Disagree Somewhat	Neither Agree nor Disagree	Agree Somewhat	Agree Totally
1	2	3	④	5

4. I regularly initiate discussions with my mate about my thoughts, opinions, and ideas.

Disagree Totally	Disagree Somewhat	Neither Agree nor Disagree	Agree Somewhat	Agree Totally
1	2	3	④	5

5. My spouse would agree that I am an affectionate person.

Disagree Totally	Disagree Somewhat	Neither Agree nor Disagree	Agree Somewhat	Agree Totally
1	2	③	4	5

6. I am sensitive to my mate's feelings and know how to respond in an appropriate, helpful way when he or she is angry, sad, hurt, or even joyful.

Disagree Totally	Disagree Somewhat	Neither Agree nor Disagree	Agree Somewhat	Agree Totally
1	2	3	④	5

Intimacy score: __19__ *out of a possible 30 points.*

6. Cooperation

1. My spouse would agree that I am an effective and respectful problem-solver.

Disagree Totally	Disagree Somewhat	Neither Agree nor Disagree	Agree Somewhat	Agree Totally
1	2	3	④	5

2. I work well with my mate on many different projects.

Disagree Totally	Disagree Somewhat	Neither Agree nor Disagree	Agree Somewhat	Agree Totally
1	2	③	4	5

3. My mate would agree that we work well together to run and keep our home and raise our children.

Disagree Totally	Disagree Somewhat	Neither Agree nor Disagree	Agree Somewhat	Agree Totally
1	2	③	4	5

4. I am good at steering arguments and disagreements to a respectful and mutually satisfying resolution.

Disagree Totally	Disagree Somewhat	Neither Agree nor Disagree	Agree Somewhat	Agree Totally
1	②	3	4	5

5. I regularly initiate discussions about future plans with my mate, and I am good at working with him or her to make sure those plans actually materialize.

Disagree Totally	Disagree Somewhat	Neither Agree nor Disagree	Agree Somewhat	Agree Totally
1	2	③	④	5

6. My mate would agree that I consistently take him or her and the family into consideration when setting my schedule and planning how to spend my time and energy.

Disagree Totally	Disagree Somewhat	Neither Agree nor Disagree	Agree Somewhat	Agree Totally
1	2	③	4	5

Cooperation score: __19__ *out of a possible 30 points.*

7. Joy

1. I am able to marvel at God's hand in simple, everyday things.

Disagree Totally	Disagree Somewhat	Neither Agree nor Disagree	Agree Somewhat	Agree Totally
1	2	3	④	5

2. I look for opportunities to be silly and playful.

Disagree Totally	Disagree Somewhat	Neither Agree nor Disagree	Agree Somewhat	Agree Totally
①	2	3	4	5

3. I am in touch with my senses and am passionate about experiencing life through all of them.

Disagree Totally	Disagree Somewhat	Neither Agree nor Disagree	Agree Somewhat	Agree Totally
1	②	3	4	5

4. My mate would agree that I have a healthy, respectful, and engaging sense of humor.

Disagree Totally	Disagree Somewhat	Neither Agree nor Disagree	Agree Somewhat	Agree Totally
①	2	3	4	5

5. I enjoy surprises.

Disagree Totally	Disagree Somewhat	Neither Agree nor Disagree	Agree Somewhat	Agree Totally
1	2	3	4	(5)

6. I love discovering new things and exploring new places and ideas.

Disagree Totally	Disagree Somewhat	Neither Agree nor Disagree	Agree Somewhat	Agree Totally
1	2	3	4	(5)

Joyfulness score: __18__ *out of a possible 30 points.*

8. Personhood

1. I know in my heart that I am made in the image and likeness of God, and I strive to exhibit all the virtues and qualities that make me fully human (e.g., rationality, emotionality, nurturance, communicativeness, passion, creativity, wisdom).

Disagree Totally	Disagree Somewhat	Neither Agree nor Disagree	Agree Somewhat	Agree Totally
1	2	3	(4)	5

2. I know that God created my body and I am pleased with the body God has given me, enjoy caring for my body and health, and feel competent with the use of my body.

Disagree Totally	Disagree Somewhat	Neither Agree nor Disagree	Agree Somewhat	Agree Totally
1	2	3	(4)	5

3. I am not embarrassed or squeamish about my bodily functions.

Disagree Totally	Disagree Somewhat	Neither Agree nor Disagree	Agree Somewhat	Agree Totally
1	2	3	(4)	5

4. I am a strong and confident person fully capable of expressing my needs and wants in every area of my life.

Disagree Totally	Disagree Somewhat	Neither Agree nor Disagree	Agree Somewhat	Agree Totally
1	2	3	4	(5)

5. While I acknowledge that there are real differences between men and women, I do not think of men and women as different species who cannot understand each other. Rather, I understand the Church's teaching that being "masculine" or "feminine" refers to living out all of the virtues that make me human through the body God has given me.

Disagree Totally	Disagree Somewhat	Neither Agree nor Disagree	Agree Somewhat	Agree Totally
1	2	3	4	(5)

6. I know that I am a son or daughter of the Most High God. I understand the privileges to which that entitles me (in this life and the next) and I accept the responsibilities (living a moral, God-centered life) that accompany my God-given nobility.

Disagree Totally	Disagree Somewhat	Neither Agree nor Disagree	Agree Somewhat	Agree Totally
1	2	3	4	(5)

Personhood score: __27__ *out of a possible 30 points.*

Summary of Scores

Write your scores for each section in the blanks below and then total the scores to determine the degree to which you demonstrate Infallible Loving in your marriage today.

_14_ Self-Donative Love   _19_ Intimacy

_13_ Responsibility   _19_ Cooperation

_23_ Faith   _18_ Joy

_17_ Respect   _27_ Personhood

69

Total score: _152_ out of a possible 240 points.

Scoring Key

220–240: Infallible Lover. You have what it takes to be an exceptional lover in and out of the bedroom. While your sexual relationship can continue to improve with ongoing specific, open discussions about your sexual likes and dislikes, the foundation of mutual respect and genuine love is there to make these conversations comfortable and fruitful.

190–219: Thoughtful Lover. You appreciate the specialness of your intimate relationship but sometimes struggle to appreciate the spiritual depth of sexual intimacy. You know sex is meaningful but aren't always sure how to practically connect with everything you may have heard it could be. You try to be attentive to your spouse, but sometimes other influences inside and outside you distract you and cause you to not be as present as you might like to be. Being more mindful of the one or two areas where you scored the lowest will help you shore up the foundation upon which to build a truly loving, healthy, whole, and holy sexual life.

165–189: Casual Lover. You may think of sex more as meaningful recreation than something with greater spiritual significance. Your view of sex is only casually connected to the greater spiritual significance afforded it by Infallible Lovers. Regardless of your sexual history, your views of sex are largely rooted in eroticism. You recognize that marriage makes sex "special" in some way, but may be hard-pressed to meaningfully articulate why. Regarding your relationship, you may tend to neglect the many opportunities for demonstrating love and intimacy throughout the day and instead focus too much on sex as the primary means of maintaining a connection between you and your mate. Unfortunately, the strength of your sexual connection may decrease as well, as missed opportunities for intimacy undermine your or your mate's desire for intercourse. Concentrate on the virtues that you scored lowest in and pay close attention to the sections in this book that focus on connecting your sexuality to the divine spark from which Holy Sex draws its power. Faithful counseling may help you move more rapidly toward becoming an Infallible Lover.

164 or Lower: Student of Eroticism. You probably have a very difficult time thinking of sex in spiritual terms at all. At best, you may view sex as a wonderfully fun thing to do that is primarily about sensuality and secondarily about relationship. At worst, you may think that sex is entirely too naughty, perverse, or at least base to merit spiritual consideration. In either case, sex is more of an activity than an expression of the self. The whole idea that sex conveys important spiritual realities or virtues may seem odd, absurd, or even offensive. You need to reckon with the fact that your views of sex have little to do with sex at all and are really based almost exclusively on observations or experiences of eroticism. You can still become an Infallible Lover, but it will take real humility and a commitment to learn about many things you have ignored or dismissed out of hand. Counseling may be useful to help you reconnect your dis-integrated sexuality to your humanity. Contact the Pastoral Solutions Institute (*www.exceptionalmarriages.com*) for more information.

How Did You Do?

Having completed the preceding quiz, you have a better sense of the strengths and weaknesses in your own sexuality. But possibly, as you read through the items, you had some questions. For example: you may have wondered what some of the items had to do with sexuality. Or, perhaps, if you scored lower in one section or another, you may be curious about how you could increase the presence of that trait in your life.

THE EIGHT STEPS TO INFALLIBLE LOVING

Fear not, intrepid reader, for the best is yet to come. In the next portion of the chapter, we're going to answer each of those questions. Let's go back to the beginning of the quiz and work our way through this outline one step at a time.

1. Self-Donative Love

The term "self-donation" figures prominently in the writings of Pope John Paul II when he talks about marriage and family life. Self-donation is love, but it is a special kind of love that empowers us to use our bodies, minds, and souls to work for the good of others, even while being mindful of our own, God-given dignity.

The person who is accomplished at self-donation has the ability to make others feel loved and attended to. He knows how to be loving (defined as "working for the good of another") even when he doesn't feel like it; even if the person being loved doesn't always deserve such generosity. In short, the self-donative person is a cheerful, thoughtful, loving, and generous servant. And yet, he is able to do this without being a doormat, without allowing himself to be victimized or unreasonably taken advantage of by others. He is able to balance these two things (generosity and the need to set boundaries) because he is guided by a deep sense of his own God-given worth, and the God-given worth of those put in his path.

Obviously, the ability to practice self-donative love is extremely important in the sexual sphere. Self-donation prepares a person to do whatever is best for himself and his lover at any given moment, whether that means giving all of oneself, or holding something back because the time is not yet right to give it (just as God, who is completely self-donative, does not reveal all of himself and all of the blessings he wants to give us at once). Perhaps even more important, a truly healthy, Christian sexuality is founded on the belief that lovemaking is the fullest expression of how well, lovingly, and respectfully the lovers care for one another — not just in the bedroom, but all day long. If you would care to increase the presence of self-donation in your marriage and especially in your sexual relationship, try the following recommendations.

Exercise
DEVELOP A MARITAL MISSION STATEMENT

To help facilitate self-donation in yourself and your mate, I recommend the use of a marital mission statement. Essentially, this is a list of the virtues you wish to emphasize in your relationship and a plan for practicing those virtues. For example, if you wanted to emphasize (1) faith, (2) joy, (3) respect, and (4) service in your home, you might make sure to (1) "pray together as a couple for fifteen minutes a day," (2) "be more open to new experiences (sexual and otherwise) my mate suggests," (3) "speak respectfully when we make requests of one another," (4) "look for ways to help each other out without being asked."

A marital mission statement is one way to remind each other that every moment carries with it an invitation to become a better person and a more attentive lover. It helps couples see that there are bigger things at stake than "what I feel like doing at the moment." This is an important skill for marriage, as it directly affects our ability to put the needs of another over our own feelings. In fact, it is exactly this ability to put the needs of another over our immediate wants or feelings that makes self-donation so important to sexuality. (For more specific assistance on how to develop your own marital mission statement, see my book *For Better . . . FOREVER! The Catholic Guide to Lifelong Marriage.*)

Practice Generosity

I encourage couples to look for little ways to serve each other all day long. Some practical ways to do this are to look for little messes to clean up whether you made them or not, or volunteer to do those tasks that are tiring to your mate, or offer to be on-point with the kids. Each of these is a simple way to be on the lookout for opportunities to serve your spouse.

While this may seem only tangentially related to sexuality, we need to remember that sexuality is really an expression of our whole character. Since this is the case, the ability to have a loving, attentive, respectful, servant's heart is the hallmark of a truly godly lover, both in and out of the bedroom. In fact, one recent psychological study documented that the degree to which a married couple reported their sexual relationship to be satisfying (i.e., both respectful and pleasurable) was directly related to how well the couple felt they worked together to complete housekeeping and childrearing tasks.

Another way to encourage generosity in your marriage is to work hard to see the truth, goodness, and beauty in all the things your mate finds true, good, and beautiful. If you like art, Mexican food, monster truck rallies, football, ballet, or the color yellow and I don't, I could pick on you for liking those things — or at the very least, hide in the basement when you attempt to pursue those interests. Alternatively, I could be generous to you and try to foster some appreciation for those things, mainly because I love you and I want you to feel that you can share the things that are important to you with me. I may never learn to have the same appreciation for the things you enjoy, but because I regularly and generously participate in the activities and interests you have, you will feel like I respect you, I am interested in your life, and I truly want to be your friend. Compare this to those marriages where husbands and wives have best friends who are not their mates (because "My wife can't stand when I talk about..." or, "My husband would rather set himself on fire than join me in...") and you begin to understand the importance generosity plays in helping a couple celebrate a truly intimate marriage.

As you practice these suggestions, you'll come to a deeper appreciation that the most important thing you can do is not satisfy yourself, but find satisfaction in working for the good of those around you. This will make you a more generous, thoughtful lover, and inspire your mate to be more generous and thoughtful as well.

Exercise

MAKE SURE MARRIAGE AND FAMILY IS YOUR PRIORITY

We all struggle to balance the many responsibilities that tug at us every day. But true self-donation requires us to first attend to the people God has directly entrusted to our care. We cannot give the best of ourselves to friends, co-workers, and community, and give the leftovers to our families. This is the antithesis of the self-donation expected of a married person.

To maintain your priority for your marriage and balance all the other responsibilities in your life, use the following formula as a guide.

1. Think of a week in the recent past when you could say that your family was functioning at its best. (Marriage solid. Kids basically compliant. Good rapport all around). Now ask yourself, "How much time did we spend playing, talking, and working together that week?" The answer to this question is the amount of time your marriage and family requires to run well.

2. There is a line that exists between fulfilling our obligation to give our employers a full day's work and our need to inflate ourselves by making the most money or being the best-loved employee. How much time and energy does it take to give your employer a full day's work (and meet your financial needs) without stepping over that line to the point that you are working for wealth and your own glorification? That is the amount of time to give to your work.

3. Now add the two amounts of time from "1" and "2" together. This figure represents the amount of time in your week that should be devoted to your work and family. Subtract that number from the number of hours you are awake in the week. Feel free to divide

whatever is left over among friends, hobbies, and community service projects.

By using this formula, you will learn to guard the priority of your family, affording opportunities to practice self-donation to build a "community of love."

2. Responsibility
(½ cup self-discipline; ½ cup stewardship)

Responsibility is the virtue that helps us decide how best to respond to our circumstances — to conduct ourselves with dignity, to nurture the people and maintain the things God has blessed us with. Responsibility has everything to do with sexuality because it encourages us to practice self-mastery, it tells us how to treat other people with the dignity that they deserve, and it enables us to become trustworthy so that others can feel safe being vulnerable around us.

To increase the amount of responsibility you display in your family, practice self-discipline. Work hard to stop pouting or being irritable when you can't have what you want. Set goals and work toward them. Look for opportunities to serve your family and make their lives easier (and ask your children to do the same). Take up the old spiritual discipline of fasting as a way to increase your capacity to delay gratification.

Another part of responsibility is stewardship; taking good care of the things that are in your dominion (keeping your house, grounds, finances, and car in order). Stewardship is not about keeping your things clean and well-maintained so that they can look like they belong in a museum. Stewardship is really about keeping things clean and maintained so that others will feel comfortable using them. If your family lives in fear of sitting on the couches or spending a penny of your hard-earned money or if they miss you because you're so busy cleaning and classifying your whoopee-cushion collection, you are offending stewardship because you're sending the message that things are more important than people. Of course, this affects sexuality, because if your mate thinks that you value your things more than you value him or her, how can you reasonably expect your mate to offer the kind of trust that a whole and holy sexual relationship requires? Of course, you can't.

Responsibility, defined here as a exhibiting both self-discipline and true, hospitable stewardship in all the circumstances of your life, is essential to expressing a healthy, holy sexuality.

3. Faith

Faith is absolutely essential for a whole and holy sexuality because it clarifies the ideal for Christian sexuality and provides a context for that sexuality to be expressed. The Pontifical Council for the Family's *Truth and Meaning of Human Sexuality* insists that it is impossible to enjoy the fullness of Holy Sex unless we actively keep the spiritual and moral dimensions of sexuality in mind. In fact, for the Christian, sexuality has its roots not in biology, but in the soul. Sexuality is not merely the way one body expresses itself to another; it is really the way one soulful, mindful, noble, and embodied *person* expresses himself or herself to another soulful, mindful, noble, and embodied *person.* Likewise, the Christian is called to remember that the act of lovemaking is not merely an expression of love between a husband and wife, but rather, it is a physical sign of the intense, all-consuming passion with which God himself seeks to love us (see the Song of Songs).

For Christians, sexuality is really a prayer that enables us to give ourselves to work for the good of another as well as to bring unity and new life into the world. This is why even celibate priests and religious can have a vital sexuality because true sexuality — in its broadest sense — is not so much a *genital act* as it is the act of using one's body and one's labors to bring about peace, to create new things, and to manifest God's passionate love for another. Psychologists and theologians both know that sexuality and genitality are two different but related things. We express our sexuality any time we work to build intimacy in our lives and fulfill the generative impulse through creativity, nurturing, or building up. We express our genitality when we express the human need for intimacy and generativity through intercourse. In his book *Christianity and Eros,* Orthodox theologian Paul Sherrard argues that in order to experience what I call Holy Sex — that is, sex as a spiritually transformative and grace-filled encounter between man, woman, and God — the couple must activate their sexual power, not only in lovemaking (genitality) but also in every act of service, communication, or intimacy throughout the day, so that every aspect of their lives is charged with sexual energy. In *For Better...FOREVER!* I argue that Infallible Lovers are able to experience the same sort of intimate connection whether they are in each other's arms or doing yard work together. This, of course, is not the same as saying that Holy Sex is no more exciting than scraping gum off a shoe. Infallible Lovers know how to fill almost everything they do together with as much intimacy and grace as their circumstances permit, and therefore, rather than taking their sexuality off the shelves and dusting it off once a week or so as is the practice with lesser lovers, Infallible Lovers celebrate their sexuality all day long through intimate communication and loving service.

In order to exhibit a sexuality that is founded on faith, we cannot save sexuality for the bedroom and faith for church on Sunday morning. We must be committed to living out both our sexuality and our faith in our everyday lives, and not be afraid to apply that faith to — and express our sexuality in — everything we do in the course of the day with our mate.

To that end, we must pray together with our mate, formally and informally, as well as receive the sacraments frequently, and engage in regular Bible reading and study. Beyond this, though, we must learn that prayer, just like sexuality (because both are ordered toward unity, intimacy, and generativity), is not something that we do, but rather something that we are. Prayer does not simply consist of those things I do when I am in church or holding a rosary; it is also everything I do in the course of a day from washing the dishes, to doing my paperwork, to parenting my children, to making love with my mate, *if* (1) I seek to experience God in those moments and (2) I seek to serve God in those moments.

4. Respect
(½ cup self-respect with ½ cup respect for others)

This is a big one. Having a healthy respect for oneself and others includes such qualities as modesty, as well as the ability to treat others with the dignity they deserve and the ability to set respectful limits when others accidentally or intentionally treat you in a manner that is beneath your God-given dignity. Applying respect to sexuality means that I have a good understanding of what it means to live and dress modestly (not dumpily though; see below), that I do not use others as a means to satisfy myself (either in or out of the bedroom), and I am good at setting limits with people who ask me to betray my God-given dignity. Let's take a look at each of these.

Modesty

Modesty has much more to do with one's internal attitude than it does with hemlines. The great Catholic physician and philosopher Dr. Herbert Ratner (who accomplished more good for the Church and the world in his lifetime than you or I could ever hope to) once said that a nun could be forced to walk naked down the street and still find a way to carry herself modestly, while Marilyn Monroe (or, perhaps a more contemporary example would be celebutante Paris Hilton) could walk down the street in a nun's full habit and still find a way to seem immodest.

Just as many people acquaint chastity with repression, so too many people equate modesty with dumpiness. As popular Catholic speaker Mary Beth Bonnacci wrote in an issue of *Envoy* magazine, certain people who think they are pursuing modesty "seem to fear all attraction to the opposite sex. Some women seem to make a test out of requiring men to look past their deliberately slovenly appearance to find the 'gold' of inner beauty disguised within. Personally, I don't think this is such a hot idea."

She goes on to say, "The object of modesty is to elevate the dignity of the human person. It's to demonstrate that we respect the human body as the seat of the soul, as a gift from God. We keep the sexual function of

the body private out of respect, but . . . we also show respect fo
when we dress attractively."

The upshot is that if we dress in a manner that glorifies ourselves, either
by saying, "Look at what hot stuff I am," or, "Look at how piously dumpy
I am," then we are being immodest.

Fr. Peter Stravinkas notes that modesty is a social virtue that facilitates
relationships by preventing people from either behaving (or appearing) too
shocking with each other or behaving (or appearing) too fussy with each
other. In order to practice modesty, of course, you should be sensitive to
the message you are sending by what you wear, but even more important,
you should avoid gossiping about others to make yourself feel better, more
pious, or more accomplished, and you should practice and encourage the
ability to display all your gifts and talents while avoiding the temptation
to say, "Hey, everybody, look at me!" all of the time.

Not Using Others to Satisfy Myself

Using other people is an obvious affront to both respect and Christian
sexuality. On the one hand, Christian sexuality calls us to be a generous,
attentive, respectful, loving servant to another person. On the other hand,
selfish sexuality causes us to think of ourselves as an itch that others
are expected to scratch. But few people appreciate that selfishness in the
bedroom has its roots far outside the bedroom. For instance, as you go
about your day, do you shirk your responsibilities and expect everyone
else to clean up your messes? Do you expect others to do for you what
you are perfectly capable of doing for yourself? Do you attempt to act like
your mate's superior, giving and denying permission at will for things that
are important to them? Do you think about others primarily in terms of
how associating with them can benefit you? If you said "yes," to any of
the above, then chances are, whether you have intended to or not, you
have made your mate feel used at one time or another, and I am willing to
bet that you are experiencing the fallout form this "using" in your sexual
relationship.

Setting Limits with People Who Ask Me to Betray My God-given Dignity

Setting respectful limits with others who either treat us in demeaning ways or ask us to do things that are beneath our God-given dignity is absolutely essential to developing solid character, fostering healthy relationships, and celebrating a healthy (and holy) sexuality.

If I do not know how to set limits, then I often feel taken advantage of by people who want me to do things that are really not good for me to do. The real problem, though, is not that others take advantage of me, but that I can't say no to people because I would feel too guilty disappointing them (or alternatively, because I am too afraid of their anger). But my morality is dependent upon my ability to set limits, and my self-esteem is dependent upon how true I am to my morality.

Knowing how to set healthy limits prevents you from worrying that your spouse will take advantage of you or take you for granted in the bedroom. Without this ability, you will either too easily agree to do things in bed that make you resentful and undermine intimacy, or you will constantly hold back from your mate in an attempt to stave off every possibility that you might be taken advantage of, in which case your sex life will be governed by more rules than the tax code and will be just as joyful.

If you would like to become better at setting respectful limits in your life, please see my book *God Help Me, These People Are Driving Me Nuts! Making Peace with Difficult People* (Loyola, 2001).

5. Intimacy
(combine equal parts verbal and emotional communication)

Intimacy, the ability to express yourself verbally and emotionally, is essential for both good character and a healthy sexuality. It is your capacity for intimacy that helps others know where they stand at all times and prevents them from ever feeling used, because they know where you're coming from.

As I write in *For Better . . . FOREVER!* intimacy is to love what a depth gauge is to a body of water. A couple may say that they love each other, but whether that love is a puddle or an ocean depends upon each person's capacity for intimacy, that is, their capacity to express themselves verbally and emotionally.

There are some who believe that intimacy is gender based in that it is primarily a "female" quality. For reasons that I will explain later (hint: it has to do with complementarity of roles and the original unity of man and woman) this concept flies in the face of Church teaching. For now, suffice it to say that Jesus Christ, who was fully human, fully man, and therefore fully masculine, was capable of deep intimacy with those he loved. Scripture shows convincingly that he was a man who was completely capable of expressing both his thoughts and his emotions very well. All men (and women) would do well to follow his example.

If you would like to foster more intimacy in your relationship, challenge yourselves to consider how well you attend to each other's spiritual and emotional well-being each day. For instance, husbands and wives should both work to be as affectionate with each other as possible while retaining a sense of propriety. And husbands and wives should have at least a working knowledge of their mate's work, roles, and interests, so that they always have plenty to discuss and share. You can find more tips on expanding your intimacy in every aspect of your marital relationship in *For Better...FOREVER! A Catholic Guide to Lifelong Marriage.*

6. Cooperation

Cooperation may seem like an odd virtue to include in a discussion on sexuality, but it is really quite important. Whether you are the sort of person who knows how to work respectfully with another to solve problems and meet goals is directly related to how well you are able to work with your spouse to create a mutually satisfying sexual relationship, plan the size of your family, negotiate the frequency of lovemaking, and make it through those times of continence that Natural Family Planning requires (see chapters 10 and 15).

... struggle in this area review the chapter in *For Better ... FOREVER!* titled "The Secrets of Red Hot Loving" for tips on how to be loving even when conflict heats things up.

7. Joy

Joy, as C. S. Lewis describes it in his book *Surprised by Joy,* is really the ability to experience God in the little events of daily living. It is the ability to look at a sunset, a tree, the face of a friend, or the body of a lover and say, "God is so wonderful.... Look at all the beauty he has surrounded me with."

Of course, joy is the ability to celebrate the God-given pleasures of life. Joy is the virtue referenced in the Jewish proverb that says, "We will be held accountable before God for all the permitted pleasures that we fail to enjoy."

Joy is an important part of our sexuality. It allows us to be playful with our mate, to laugh and be silly without taking or offering offense. It allows us to celebrate in each other's arms, and even to experience lovemaking as a physical sign of how passionately God himself loves us.

To cultivate joy, look for opportunities to be playful and silly and cultivate a respectful sense of humor. Even more important, leave your comfort zone and open yourself up to sharing new experiences with your mate. Practice the following motto: "As long as it doesn't demean my personal dignity or violate my morals, sign me up!" For additional suggestions on cultivating joy in your sexual relationship, review chapters 11–13 on pleasure, foreplay, and intercourse.

8. Personhood

Personhood may sound like an odd characteristic, but it figures prominently in Pope John Paul II's writings. While it has many dimensions for our purposes, we are going to define it as encompassing the following:

1. An appreciation for what it means to be made in the image and likeness of God.

2. An acknowledgment of the goodness of the body and a respect for the spiritual meaning of the body.

3. An understanding of what it means to be a fully functioning Christian man or woman.

Whole books could be and have been written on these three things, and I cannot hope to do them justice in the short space I have available here. Nevertheless, we need to look at this quality at least briefly because it has everything to do with whether we have a healthy and holy sense of our sexuality.

To appreciate being made in the image and likeness of God is to have an understanding of what it is to be a fully functioning human being. God is the source of our unique dignity because everything that we consider about ourselves to be good comes directly from God. As C. S. Lewis put it, "[God] lends us a little of His reasoning powers and that is how we think: He puts a little of His love into us and that is how we love one another," like a little child learning to write his letters. Celebrating the fact that we are made in God's image and likeness means that each day we try to increase our capacity, our facility, with all of the virtues that make us human. Every day we look for opportunities to grow in love, creativity, intelligence, passion, joy, generosity, and all the virtues that enable us to live life as a gift. It is the ability to pursue these virtues as well as our actual pursuit of these virtues that makes us truly human.

So what does this have to do with sexuality? Everything. When I work to manifest the God-given virtues that underlie my humanity on a daily basis, I end up sanctifying my everyday life. Taking out the garbage is no longer about taking out the garbage; it becomes an opportunity for me to practice service or generosity. Likewise, when I truly understand what it is to be made in the image and likeness of God, lovemaking is not just a pleasant thing I do with my mate; it becomes an opportunity to practice all the virtues that make me human: self-donation, respect, temperance, joy, patience, a pro-life ethic, and so on. Personhood allows me to experience my sexuality as a prayer that elevates both me and my spouse and manifests

God's own love for each of us. To encourage this aspect of personhood, we need to acquaint ourselves with the works of mercy (spiritual and corporal) as well as all the virtues we receive as free and unmerited gifts at baptism (i.e., the gifts and fruits of the Holy Spirit, the cardinal virtues, and the theological virtues). We need to cultivate these virtues in our everyday lives by looking for opportunities to live them out in the simple tasks we do, and by developing the mission statement I discussed earlier (see above, p. 52). In this way, we emphasize the fact that everything we do, think, and feel, even our sexuality, has a spiritual component and spiritual ramifications.

Regarding the second point, personhood is the quality that compels me to think of my body as a gift and to acknowledge my bodily functions not as "icky" but as an integral part of the creation God pronounces to be "good" in the book of Genesis.

I recall counseling a woman who hated making love to her husband. By her own admission, her husband was a good and loving man, he was romantic and attentive, he did not demean her in any way, they did not have significant arguments, and, generally speaking, they were good friends. In other words, there was absolutely no relational justification for her lack of interest in lovemaking. So what was the problem? This woman was very uncomfortable with her body and bodily things. I asked her to write a journal entry on the topic of "what goes through your mind when you think about sex." This is an excerpt from that journal.

Sex. Ugh. I hate everything about it. I don't like being breathed on, I don't like being touched, especially on my private parts. After all, that's where I go to the bathroom from, why would I want to be touched there and why would I want to touch him there? How gross is that? And sex is so messy. I hate the squishy, icky, mess of it all. I would be happy if I never had to have sex. Why can't my husband just get over his need for sex (I guess because he's a guy — that's what guys do right?) and just concentrate on our spiritual lives?

While the woman who wrote this was an otherwise fine person who had many positive qualities and traits, this kind of thinking (separating "spiritual things" from our bodily nature) represents a serious affront to the quality of personhood and is just the sort of dualism that has been condemned as heretical since the earliest days of Christianity. Personhood is the quality that allows us to understand the spiritual nature of material things, especially our bodies. To encourage the development of personhood in this context we need to do two things. First, while being mindful of modesty, we need to not be "grossed out," shocked, or scandalized by our bodies and the things our bodies do. Scripture says, "I am fearfully and wonderfully made." We must be thankful for our bodies and all the wonderful things our bodies do, because all of those things were created by God to help our bodies function well. And God himself pronounced them good (see Genesis 1). When people are struggling with this kind of loathing of their body and physical nature, counseling is almost always indicated. Such individuals are completely resistant to their spouse's encouragement to be more sexually forthcoming because, to their minds, the real problem is that their mate is simply "oversexed." While "oversexed" mates do exist, they are not as common as one might think.

Finally, personhood means having a proper understanding of what it is to be a man or a woman. Unfortunately, this is often the least understood concept, even by faithful Catholics.

Catholics and non-Catholics alike tend to give in to the line of thinking that says "men are from Mars and women are from Venus." They say things like, "Men are rational, sexual, competitive, logical, etc. and women are nurturing, communicative, romantic, emotional." While there truly are differences between the sexes, they are not so simple as this.

The Church teaches that in the beginning God shared the *same* aspects of himself (i.e., the same sets of characteristics and virtues) with both male and female *human beings.* Genesis 1:26–28 says, "Male and female he created *them.*" As John Paul II states about the theology of the body, the fact that Adam said of Eve, "At last, this is flesh of my flesh and bone of my bone" dramatically shows that in body, mind, and soul, Eve was a being to whom Adam could relate completely. Our first parents were made of the same essential biological, psychological, emotional, and spiritual *stuff.*

At the dawn of creation, both men and women were given the ability to reason, emote, love, communicate, produce, set goals, nurture, and so on. Likewise, both men and women were called to live out *all* of these qualities to the fullest. However, based on how God created their bodies, Adam and Eve had different *styles* of applying these qualities to everyday life. So, for example, while both Adam and Eve were given the responsibility to nurture, emote, communicate, etc., God created Eve's body to *emphasize* such qualities in her life, and this emphasis was what God called "femininity." Likewise, while both Adam and Eve were given the responsibility to make plans, set goals, provide for their needs, solve problems, etc., God created Adam's body to *emphasize* such qualities in his life and this emphasis is what the Lord called "masculinity" (see *The Theology of the Body* and *Original Unity of Man and Woman: Catechesis on the Book of Genesis*, both collections of writings and talks by Pope John Paul II; see also *The Theology of the Body for Beginners* by Christopher West, and "Theology of the Body" in *The Encyclopedia of Catholic Doctrine*).

A good example of these emphases at work is how men and women practice their call to nurture young children. God ordained a woman's body to nurse her young. But even though men cannot lactate, God still requires them to be abundantly present and active in the lives of their children, just as God, Our Father, is present and active in our lives. God gave both men and women the ability to be *fully* nurturing and loving, but he ordained the sexes to express this fullness in equally valuable, yet different and complementary ways. As John Paul II teaches us, men and women must prayerfully contemplate and emphasize their bodies' unique capabilities to first understand true masculinity and femininity. Then, we must use our masculinity and femininity as the prism through which we express our full humanity.

In trying to live out what it is to be a man or woman of God, we would do well to avoid the attitudes that say things like, "Women shouldn't handle the finances because that's a man's job" and "Men aren't good at nurturing children because that's a woman's job." It is exactly this attitude that offends the generosity required of Infallible Loving (by limiting the ways a husband and wife are willing to serve each other) and flies in the face of what the Church says God originally intended when he created men and women.

If we want to experience the full, complementary meaning of masculinity and femininity, we must avoid the use of limited templates that offer a too narrow definition of manliness or womanliness (like "All men are athletic. All women like to decorate.") and instead exhibit all of the qualities God has given us to the fullest through the bodies that God has given us. In this way, we will develop a deeper appreciation for the fact that men and women are capable of many of the same things, but they will approach these tasks with a slightly different perspective and use slightly different methods. Even so, each has equal dignity in the eyes of the Lord and each brings unique gifts to every task they work on together, or independently. This will be experienced in the bedroom as a respect for each other's sexuality and the gifts that masculinity and femininity bring to the bedroom, instead of the unfair and passion-killing suspicion that claims, "Men only want one thing" and "Women never want to give it up." This may be true of men and women who are studying in the school of eroticism, but it is never true of men and women who are striving to celebrate Holy Sex and be Infallible Lovers to one another. After all, man is never more manly than when he is loving and serving woman. Woman is never more womanly than when she is loving and serving man. And the fullness of our humanity is never more beautifully expressed than when both of these realities exist at the same time.

A CONCLUSION...

Throughout this chapter, I have attempted to broaden your understanding of what it means to say that you want to experience a full, healthy, holy sexuality in your marriage. As you have seen, sexuality is about much more than "what we do with our genitals." Genitality is an important aspect of sexuality, but the authentic sexuality expressed by Holy Sex is about taking full advantage of every moment to be the best lover this moment allows you to be. Sexuality, then, is ultimately about how we communicate ourselves to others and use our bodies to work for the good of others whether that is on a one-on-one basis in marriage, or in the broader, more spiritual sense of serving the world through celibate, religious life.

If you take nothing else from this chapter, remember that "working on improving your sex life" goes far beyond expanding your repertoire of positions, packing more lingerie in the closet, or seeking out other means of heightening sensuality. Infallible Lovers may do all of these things, but they are just the beautiful and tasty icing on an already delicious cake. Rather, Infallible Lovers know that the deepest, most fulfilling, passionate, intimate, soulful sex occurs between two lovers who want to inspire each other to be the best people they can be for each other all day, and then give all of themselves to each other — body, mind, and spirit — at night.

4 CLIMBING HIGHER:
THE SEXUALITY CONTINUUM

A person first loves himself because he is carnal and sensitive to nothing but himself. Then, when he sees he cannot exist by himself, he begins to seek God by faith. . . . So in the second degree of love, man loves God for his own sake and not for God's own sake. . . . When man tastes how sweet God is, he passes to the third degree of love in which he loves God not because of his own needs, but because of God. . . . [In the fourth degree] he loves only for God's sake.

— St. Bernard of Clairvaux, *On Loving God*

So far we've discussed how Holy Sex compares with its chief competitor, eroticism, and we've explored what Infallible Lovers are made of. Next I want to illustrate the development of the Infallible Lover. This chapter will help you identify where you and your beloved are on the sexuality continuum and discover what you need to do to create a truly whole and holy sexual relationship.

What separates Infallible Lovers from all the rest? While lesser lovers bring only certain aspects of themselves to the sexual relationship, Infallible Lovers make love with every aspect of their being; their physical, mental, relational, moral, and spiritual selves are all represented in the act of lovemaking.

The sexuality continuum represents the five stages through which sexual attitudes evolve, with each stage integrating a new aspect of the person (physical, relational, mental/emotional, and spiritual) into the sexual experience. Not every person needs to go through all five stages of the sexuality continuum. Some people, because of their healthy formation, may have a "leg up" and begin a bit higher on the continuum, being naturally more able to integrate the bodily, social, mental, and spiritual dimensions of themselves with their sexuality. Regardless, once you have found your starting place on the *sexuality continuum* you'll tend to proceed through these stages in order.

Your growth toward Holy Sex and Infallible Loving reflects growth in all the virtues we discussed in the previous chapter, helping you become not just a better lover, but a more competent, loving, lovable, responsible *person* who is capable of regulating healthy boundaries and achieving real intimacy in every area of your life.

THE FIVE STAGES OF SEXUAL ADVANCEMENT (FROM AUNT MCGILLICUDDY'S ANTIQUE URN SCHOOL TO HOLY SEX)

This chapter will review the attitudes toward sex of persons at each of the five stages and illustrate how each stage evolves into the next.

Stage One: The Negative Materialists (a.k.a. Aunt McGillicuddy's Antique Urn School)

Sex is really very overrated. People talk about how great sex is, but I don't think it's all that great. Mostly, I just do it to keep my husband happy. The only thing that really makes sex special is that it's procreative. I don't tend to think of sex as something you "enjoy" per se. Let's face it. It's kind of icky. Besides, there are just so many ways to fall into sexual sin that I think you really need to be careful.

The Negative Materialists are the folks I referred to earlier as Aunt McGillicuddy's Antique Urn School of human sexuality. Rather than using the power of their sexuality in good, true, and beautiful ways, they fear it and treat it with contempt or, at best, grudging respect.

Negative Materialists focus on the body as a *thing* — and an undesirable thing at that — which has little or no spiritual usefulness. This is ironic, because people in this category tend to hijack religious ideas to justify their pathology. In fact, in the opinion of many people in this group, the body is something so corrupted that it's best viewed as an enemy.

Every good lie contains a grain of truth. Negative Materialists are correct that the sexual urge is often inappropriately expressed and that sex has caused a lot of hurt in the world. But as Msgr. Ronald Knox wrote about Jansenism, the Negative Materialists are so hag-ridden by their hyperactively paranoid sense of sin, they forget about the greater truth: the grace of confession and the gifts of God's mercy, healing, and love. They are like a child who is so afraid of falling that he never even tries to ride the bicycle he got for his birthday. Or, to use a more scriptural analogy, they are like the man in the parable of the talents who buried his treasure for fear of losing it (Matt. 25:14–30).

The Aunt McGillicuddy view is most often held by people who have some emotional trauma in their histories or were raised in a severely punitive environment. Because sex is viewed as something dangerous, and potentially victimizing, the Negative Materialist is usually a very cautious, fearful lover who gets little personal pleasure from intercourse or perhaps even affection in general. Some Negative Materialists, like the Manicheans who fascinated St. Augustine before his conversion to Christianity, are so uncomfortable about their bodies that they don't like to think of them at all, preferring to emphasize their spiritual nature. They may appear to others to be in spiritual overdrive as they run from intimacy with real, living, breathing humans, preferring to be alone with their deep spiritual thoughts and pious practices. I'm not saying that piety is a bad thing. Piety, expressed appropriately (that is, expressed incarnationally, through relationship), is a healthy thing that leads to deeper intimacy with God and others. But the Negative Materialists hijack piety as an excuse for not having the time, energy, or desire for intimacy with mere mortals.

In the worst case, and somewhat paradoxically, some Negative Materialists may actually develop an unhealthy and potentially illicit obsession with sex, due to their constant attempts to deny the sexual aspects of their humanity; many so-called "sex addicts" fall into this latter category of Negative Materialism. Individuals who find themselves struggling with sexual compulsions often try to amputate their sexuality from their respectable selves only to find that, since sexuality is an intimate part of their humanity, their sexuality nearly forces itself to be expressed in many less than respectable ways. The harder they attempt to repress their urges, the stronger and stranger the compulsions become. We will examine the issue of sexual addiction later on. For now, let's deal with the garden variety Negative Materialist — that is, the one who loathes the body and sex but hasn't begun indulging in the dark side of eroticism.

For the Negative Materialists to advance to the next, healthier stage on the continuum, they will need to reckon with the goodness of the body and sensuality. Counseling may be indicated to help couples overcome the false beliefs about the body and sexuality that plague their lives. Learning more about the godly intention of the body, sexuality, and sensuality, for instance, by delving into Pope John Paul II's Theology of the Body will also be helpful. *The Theology of the Body for Beginners* by Christopher West is a good place to start. But education might not be enough. For many Negative Materialists, the issue is not ignorance, but woundedness. Their punitive childhoods or sexual wounding causes their psyches to be unable to process the Theology of the Body in any meaningful, practical way. Persons who hold the Negative Materialist view would do well to seek the help of a faithful counselor schooled in the clinical applications of the Theology of the Body to help them overcome the wounds — wounds that prevent them from experiencing the goodness of their body in general and their sexual self in particular.

Stage Two: The Positive Materialists

"We've always had a pretty adventurous sex life," said Gary. "Rhonda has never shied away from anything. Back in college, she even fooled around with some attractive girls in her sorority. I've been really lucky with her. Our sex life has been amazing. We've used lots of different toys and had a lot of pretty wild experiences. Like I said, things have always been good. But lately, Rhonda hasn't been herself. She's pushing me away. We used to have sex at least every day — sometimes two or three times. Now, she acts like she doesn't want anything to do with me. I don't know what the hell she wants."

Like the McGillicuddys before them, Positive Materialists also believe that the body is a *thing* that has little — if any — spiritual value, *but* they believe that sensuality is good, and they celebrate it as such. Since sex is all about pleasure and sensuality, the Positive Materialist believes that anything pleasurable must be good.

Spiritually speaking, Positive Materialists break down into three categories: (1) those who have no spiritual life and merely revel in raw sexuality (hedonists); (2) those who are suspicious of spiritual things because they believe that to be "spiritual" or "religious" you must also be sexually self-punishing; and (3) those who celebrate a kind of "low church gnostic" spirituality that confuses being sensual with being spiritual and believes that the body can do whatever feels good as long as the mind occupies itself with "mystical things." Churchgoing Positive Materialists tend to be the "God wants me to be happy" folks who genuinely don't get all the fuss about who is sleeping with whom as long as it involves two consenting whatevers. The grain of truth in this big lie is that God does want us to be happy. But Positive Materialists don't know — or conveniently ignore — that authentic happiness is a life founded upon meaningfulness, intimacy, and virtue and not mere sensuality. That, by the way, is not just a Catholic assertion, but a psychological fact, as the work of University of Pennsylvania positive psychology maven Dr. Martin Seligman demonstrates (especially in his book *Authentic Happiness*).

Many Positive Materialists are either alums of the Aunt McGillicuddy School, or children of those who were active in that school's PTA, who later broke free of the obsessive-compulsive trap of Negative Materialism by asserting the goodness of the physical sensations of sexuality.

To be fair, this position represents the very beginning of seeing the body — and the human person — as a good thing. But Positive Materialism is still a fairly shallow philosophy of sex. It inhibits true intimacy by placing "exciting sensations" over meaningful relationships and confusing mere copulation with real love. Many married couples I've counseled at this stage have little understanding — if any at all — of how to be friends to each other but believe their relationship to be secure because, as Gary said in the example above, "we used to have sex at least every day — sometimes two or three times."

Positive Materialists can't rely on the fire of their intimacy to enliven their lovemaking, so they may become dependent on kinky sex toys or "exotic" sexual practices like "swinging" or milder forms of sado-masochistic sex to keep things "interesting." Though a couple finds the novelty of such experiences fun at first, these same experiences eventually undermine the spiritual core of a marriage. The great irony is that most of these couples aren't even conscious of the spiritual core of their marriage, but as it begins rotting away, a wife may complain that she no longer feels "special" to her husband and begin to see herself as "just another way my husband relieves himself." For his part, a husband who starts out as a gung-ho, Positive Materialist ("Come on, honey, have sex with other men while I watch. It'll be great!") may eventually come to mourn the loss of a wife who "accidentally" fell in love with a sex partner she had while the couple was swinging. Or he may complain that his wife "would rather spend time with her vibrator than she would with me."

As we discovered with the Negative Materialists, within every good lie there is a grain of truth. Couples are right to celebrate the goodness of their sensuality and to engage in free and pleasurable sexual play with each other. But when human sexuality is reduced to mere eroticism, it's only a matter of time before self-esteem suffers and relationships collapse. The person who wishes to move to the next stage of sexual integration must reckon with the fact that truly fulfilling sex is driven primarily not by sensuality but by intimacy, which can be fully expressed only in the context of an exclusive, committed relationship in which healthy vulnerability and the beginnings of real love can be nurtured. Couples at this stage would do well to use the mission statement exercise described earlier (see above, p. 52) as a way to learning that there is deeper meaning in every aspect of life — especially the sexual life. Counseling may also help these individuals to overcome their tendency to treat people as objects and to heal any wounding from their overindulgence in eroticism. A basic education in the Theology of the Body would help this couple understand the relational nature of the person, and counseling would help them develop the skills necessary for authentic intimacy.

Stage Three: The Interpersonal Stage
(When "Relationship Sex" Starts to Look Good)

The next stage, "The Interpersonal Stage," represents the sexual attitudes held by most average couples in basically happy marriages.

"Jerry and I have a good sex life," says Theresa of her relationship with her husband of nine years. "We always try to find ways to keep both our relationship and our lovemaking fresh, and we're very comfortable with each other. If we struggle with anything, it's too little energy and too little time. It's hard to figure out a way to insulate ourselves from all the chaos of our lives, and sometimes that has a negative effect on our sex drives. We certainly don't love each other any less — it's just tough to find the balance."

Couples in the Interpersonal Stage think of lovemaking as "a beautiful and important" thing to do, something that brings two people together. At its best, the Interpersonal Stage serves as the beginning point of meaningful, intimate sex. It allows the husband and wife to set boundaries that protect their dignity, prevent them from treating each other as objects, and still allow the couple to enjoy a pleasurable and somewhat varied sex life within those boundaries.

This is also the first stage of sexuality where children are not seen as either a justification for sex (as with the Negative Materialists) or a threat to the sensuality desired by the Positive Materialists. Rather, lovers at the Interpersonal Stage begin to see children as a real blessing to the relationship that serves both as a sign of the love and commitment between the couple and as an invitation to the couple to become more selflessly loving. This is the first stage that really begins to wrestle with what Catholics call "responsible parenthood." That is, this is the first stage at which couples are mature enough to have at least a rudimentary sense of the need to balance the joy of bringing new life into the world with the need to provide a loving, safe, faithful environment in which that life can grow.

There tend to be two drawbacks to this stage. The first is that an unde-sirable side effect of the healthy boundary-setting is often the politicization of sexual relations. For example, a couple may have arguments over cer-tain sexual acts, which are perfectly permissible from an objective moral perspective, but make one partner feel "less equal" than the other. Oral stimulation during foreplay and sexual positions where the man enters the woman from behind are two common examples of this. Another is that of the couple who argues about how much sex is a "fair" amount when a husband and wife have differing ideas about the frequency of lovemaking.

The temptation for many couples at the Interpersonal Stage is to deal with these problems as sexual issues. But trying to solve these problems head-on will only make them worse, because they are *not* primarily sexual problems; they are *sexual manifestations* of the way this couple relates to each other in every other aspect of their relationship. The only way to completely resolve these "sexual problems" is to pursue deeper intimacy and vulnerability in the relationship overall, which will help the couple overcome the self-protective tendencies that stand between them and real passion. Without taking this frightening step, the marriage, and in turn the sexual relationship, will stagnate.

Research by Dr. John Gottman suggests that couples in the happiest marriages maintain a 20:1 ratio of positive to negative interactions across the relationship and a 5:1 ratio of positivity to negativity when in con-flict. My own clinical observations reveal that the comparatively high rate of supportive, encouraging, loving, thoughtful, affirming comments and actions as compared to criticizing, complaining, nagging, and blam-ing behaviors among these couples helps build the trust and vulnerability required for truly intimate Holy Sex.

The second difficulty of this stage is that since lovemaking is still pri-marily viewed as a pleasant (and somewhat important) *thing to do,* it tends to be placed at the bottom of the pile of other important things to do. Exhaustion and stress may be regularly allowed to jeopardize the couple's sexual relationship. If such a couple isn't careful, what was once warm, safe, pleasurable "relationship sex" can quickly turn into frustrating "I'm-too-tired-for" sex. This is really the first couple on the sexuality continuum that can benefit directly from instruction (rather than needing both instruction and counseling) in the Theology of the Body. This is possible because such a couple already has at least a basic sense of the goodness of the body and the fact that their bodies were designed for relationship — not just sensuality. Education in the Theology of the Body will help this couple realize the deeper, divine significance of their sexual love. It will also help the couple begin to connect, in at least a basic way, with the mystical dimensions of their sexual relationship. Praying *together* — especially with the specific intention that God would teach them to be better lovers to each other — will also be especially helpful to the couple who is on the cusp of learning to love with a passion that goes beyond the feelings they can generate for one another. Couples at this stage also tend to struggle with making time for all aspects of their marriage — not just the sexual relationship. Even though the marriage may be basically harmonious, it may lack a depth of intimacy that a truly soulful sexual relationship requires. Couples at the interpersonal stage would benefit from the exercises presented later in this book that foster greater social intercourse — the ability to achieve greater intimacy from the day-to-day relationship.

Finally, while it isn't as necessary for couples at this stage as it is with couples at the previous stages on the sexuality continuum, counseling can help couples at the interpersonal stage stop taking each other and their sexual relationship for granted and give them additional tools to build the deeper intimacy that will be required for them to move to the next stage on the continuum.

Stage Four : The Humanistic Stage
("Sex Isn't Something We Do; It's Something We Are")

Deborah and Phillip, married twenty-two years, have busy lives and are the parents of four children. Even so, they share what they describe as a fabulous sex life. "I don't understand my friends who tell me that their lovemaking is either flat or nonexistent," says Deborah. "Maybe we're just lucky, but the spark Phillip and I had at the start of our relationship is still there. In fact, it's more like lightning now. We know each other so well and have been through so much together, I don't see how the spark couldn't have grown. There is no one on earth who would know how to please me half as well as Phillip — in or out of bed." She gave a coy smile. *"And I know he'd say the same about me."*

At the Humanistic Stage, the couple is aware of the close connection between generous service, deep intimacy, and attentive loving in all aspects of the marriage *and* great sex in the bedroom (or any other room). The couple understands — on an *experiential* level (rather than merely an intellectual level like couples at the Interpersonal Stage) — that *sex is a language* spoken by one body and soul to another. While, for less-than-infallible lovers, sex represents something they *do,* sex for these couples is something they *are.* Lovemaking is seen as the most profound expression of the mutual service the couple gives to each other all day, every day. This is the first couple on the continuum that has an experiential understanding of the idea that when they make love, their bodies are speaking a language to each other that goes beyond words and proclaims, "Look how well we love one another — even our bodies work for each other's good!"

Practically speaking, this results in the politics and scorekeeping being removed from the bedroom (it has also been excised from the marriage in general). Because this couple's personal, dignity-protecting boundaries are now being internalized, they no longer require as many external rules to protect their integrity. As long as a sexual act respects the exclusivity of the bond and doesn't violate objective moral values, it will be acceptable to both the husband and wife — and enjoyed thoroughly.

Likewise, while couples lower down on the continuum tend to lose lovemaking in the list of other "things" they have to do, the Humanistic couple would never think of neglecting their sexual relationship. For them, to make love is to reenact their marriage ceremony, to physically renew their wedding vows, and to celebrate a ritual that symbolizes everything they are to one another. This couple does not view lovemaking as an energy-draining performance, or another "nice thing to do" that — unfortunately — they no longer have the time for. They see it as a life-giving reality in which they assert the strength of their bond and the depth of their mutual, generous service, and from which they draw strength to deal with those aspects of their lives (like work and social commitments) that are less fascinating than their relationship.

The Humanistic couple seeks to give as much priority and respect to their sex lives as they did to their wedding day. For example, almost every wedding is the result of months of careful preparation, and when the wedding day comes, most brides and grooms are exhausted — emotionally and physically — from all their labors. But, remarkably, in spite of all the exhaustion, no bride or groom ever calls his or her intended the day of the wedding and recommends putting it off. A wedding *might* be postponed for some catastrophe, but it would never be delayed simply because the couple was "too tired" or "too stressed" to bother with it today. Because this couple has the experiential understanding of sex as a re-creation of their wedding day and a celebration of everything they are to one another, they place the same priority on their lovemaking as they did their original wedding day.

The Humanistic Stage represents the first taste of the fullness of Holy Sex, when a couple has matured enough as lovers to bring their physical, mental, emotional, and relational, as well as moral and spiritual selves to their lovemaking. Sex at this level is certainly not always acrobatic, but it doesn't need to be, because it is always *passionate*. For the couple at this stage, lovemaking is an *intentional expression* of the deep friendship and intimacy they share. In light of this, sometimes Infallible Lovers may make love even when they are not initially physically desirous, because expressing desire is less important than expressing true love (their willingness to work for the good of each other). Pushing through lack of desire at this stage is different from the behavior of the Negative Materialist, who often just puts up with sex and counts the minutes till it's over. Where the Negative Materialist experiences both a duty-bound sexuality and the resentment that comes from making imprudent sacrifices for the sake of sex, lovers at the Humanistic Stage experience deeper intimacy and joy for having pushed themselves to be more sexually generous to each other. This is because the positivity expressed throughout the relationship makes the husband and wife want to be everything they can be for one another and rejoices in being able to return the love being offered so freely and generously in every other aspect of their lives together.

In sum, lovemaking at the Humanistic Stage and beyond is a wedding banquet that both husband and wife feel privileged to attend, regardless of their present physical or emotional state of being. It's a symbol of all the good things they represent to each other, and a reenactment of their promise to love one another in sickness and health, wealth and poverty, good times and bad, stress or no stress, sleep or no sleep, from this day forward, until death do them part.

It is curious, then, that some couples, as they approach the Humanistic Stage, encounter what Dr. Pepper Schwartz in *Peer Marriage* refers to as an "incest taboo" to lovemaking. In essence, the couple's relationship advances to the point where day-to-day life is so good, the marital friendship is so deep, and the couple is so intimate that — counterintuitively — sex no longer seems an appropriate way for them to relate to each other. Dr. Schwartz merely describes this phenomenon and offers no explanation for it, but since this "incest taboo" is not universally experienced by couples in the Humanistic Stage and higher, I believe that the determining factor is the attitudes the couple had about sex to begin with.

For all our claims to be a sexually liberated society, most people, thanks to our obsession with eroticism, still think of sex in negative terms. People talk about having sex as "being bad" or "getting nasty." But as a husband and wife approach becoming Infallible Lovers, there is little that is bad about themselves or their relationship, so the negative connotation of "being bad" no longer applies. In other words, since the couple gets along so well and there is no reason to ever "be nasty" *toward* each other, there is likewise no longer any congruent way to "get nasty" *with* each other. Dr. Schwartz observes that some couples try to get around this by giving themselves permission to *pretend* to "be bad" when it comes to their sex lives. But this is patently unhealthy from a psychological perspective, because it uses a defense mechanism called "compartmentalization" or "splitting": the person acts one way in one context and another way in a different context. This defense mechanism falls under the "Major Image Distorting" category (read: "Damn unhealthy") on the Defensive Functioning Scale in the *American Psychiatric Association's Diagnostic and Statistical Manual of Mental Disorders.*

The only psychologically congruent way to resolve the "incest taboo" is to see that sex was never the problem. Rather, the *metaphor* the person was using for sex was problematic. As we saw earlier, eroticism — because it is sex cut loose from true, working-for-the-good-of-each-other love — *can* be "bad" or "dirty" because it stimulates the body without respect for the soul. But eroticism and Holy Sex are two completely different things. Sex at the Humanistic Stage is never bad or dirty, because while it may involve intensely erotic elements, it also enables the couple to honor the godly nature of both husband and wife.

The couple at this stage struggling with the "incest taboo" would benefit from counseling that could help them evaluate the cognitive distortions and faulty beliefs that are clogging up the pipeline between their marital love and respect and the passionate sexuality that would otherwise be expected to flow from it. Regardless, all couples at this stage will benefit from more time to let the intimacy and respect they are cultivating in their day-to-day relationship seep into the sexual dimensions of their relationship. Moving to the next stage is more about seasoning and maturing than it is about checking off the box next to certain relational or developmental tasks. That said, all couples at this stage will benefit from continuing to foster their prayer life, specifically their prayer life around the intention of being better lovers to each other in and out of the bedroom. They can also delve more deeply into the Theology of the Body and other resources as a way of learning more about the power of sex to physically reveal God's own love for the husband and wife.

Stage Five: Holy Sex
("Lovemaking as a Spiritually Active Way
to Connect with the Divine")

"For us," says George, "sex is a kind of prayer. When we make love, Veronica and I not only work to give ourselves to each other, but we try to use our lovemaking as a way to understand how God is reaching out to each one of us." Veronica agrees, "Looking at our physical relationship this way has added a whole new dimension. Things were always good between us. But now, it's unbelievable. I don't know exactly how to put it, except to say that it's like the difference between singing a song, and becoming the song."

The *Janus Report on Sexual Behavior* states that spiritual people have more satisfying sex lives because they "pay more attention to the mystic and symbolic dimensions of one's sexuality." Here you will see why this is true. Holy Sex distinguishes itself from all the other stages by two remarkable qualities: Lovemaking as an Experience of God, and Lovemaking as a Path to Personal Growth.

Lovemaking as an Experience of God

Other couples may instinctively cry out, "Oh my God!" at the height of passion, but couples practicing Holy Sex really mean it. Lovemaking *is* a religious experience, and not just metaphorically speaking. Beyond simply honoring the goodness of human love in its most generous forms as Humanistic couples do, the highest level of exceptional sexuality emboldens a couple to understand how God himself relates to us through our sexuality. The specific ways a couple experiences this revelation may differ slightly depending upon their understanding of God and their faith tradition, but all couples practicing Holy Sex know that God is there and that he is revealing himself in a powerful way.

Earlier I quoted C. S. Lewis, who once wrote, "[God] lends us a little of His reasoning powers and that is how we think: He puts a little of His love into us and that is how we love one another." The same is true of our sexuality. God enjoys his own "sexuality," and because he is generous, he shares that sexuality — or to put it somewhat more precisely, his uniting and creative nature — with us. Some readers may be appalled by what must seem to be a hopeless anthropomorphism on my part. But when I refer to God's "sexuality," I don't mean it in the physical way we humans understand it. Rather, God's "sexuality" is expressed in the joy God "experiences" by loving all things, uniting all things, and creating all things. What we mortals refer to as our "sexuality" is the *power* God "lends us" to join him in loving, uniting, and creating both on a physical level (through lovemaking that leads to children) and on a spiritual level (through lovemaking that strengthens the unity of the couple and actualizes their values, ideals, and goals).

The most exceptional lovers understand this, and as a result they experience their lovemaking not only as self-revelation, but as divine revelation.

Lovemaking as a Path to Personal Growth

Like the Humanistic couples before them, those husbands and wives who practice Holy Sex see lovemaking as a physical expression of all that is good in their marriage. But even more important, they understand their sexuality as a powerful tool that can be used to pursue personal growth and sanctification. We'll explore this more in depth when we look at the Second Power of Holy Sex, but let me give you a brief introduction to this idea now.

The deepest levels of emotional, relational, and spiritual growth require you to embrace vulnerability — the willingness to have your weaknesses exposed so that you can be made whole. There are few instances in life when you are more vulnerable than when you are making love with your soul mate. This vulnerability can be intimidating for couples further down the sexuality continuum who protect themselves from it by setting up arbitrary rules based more upon gut-level senses than on any objective moral standard. Couples who celebrate Holy Sex, on the other hand, are exhilarated by the vulnerability they experience in the arms of their beloved because they understand the healing and transformative power that accompanies loving vulnerably. For instance:

Christianne is the mother of five children, each by cesarean section. The scars on her abdomen made her extremely self-conscious, especially during lovemaking, but initially, she was too embarrassed to share this with her husband. When she finally confessed the shame she felt over her appearance, her husband said with — she told me — unmistakable sincerity, "You are so beautiful. Each one of those marks is a gift, given to me by a woman who loves me enough to bear my children."

Any woman who has ever borne children will understand how deeply that man's words touched his wife. By exposing herself fully, body and soul, to her husband's love, she not only learned to accept her appearance, but to celebrate it. The very scars she once saw as a disfigurement are now experienced by her as "marks of honor" (her words) which tell the story of her and her husband's life-giving love.

Sex has an immense power to challenge every emotional, relational, and spiritual boundary a person has. To rise to these challenges with grace, dignity, and even passion is the goal and privilege of those couples aspiring to and living out the ideals of Holy Sex. In fact, there is a spiritual and perhaps even eternal benefit to embracing the vulnerability experienced through exceptional lovemaking, as we'll discuss later. Holy Sex challenges shame and deepens our vulnerability to our mate and to God.

IN A NUTSHELL

In this chapter, we've explored the five stages through which men and women evolve to become Infallible Lovers. In this chapter, you've seen that with each stage, the lovers bring a new dimension of themselves to lovemaking. First the lover must learn to see his or her body as a good and delightful thing, praising God, like the psalmist, that each one of us is "fearfully and wonderfully made." Next, the lover must integrate his or her social/relational self, learning that while sensuality is an important part of lovemaking, it is the intimacy that comes from an exclusive, committed, lifelong, fruitful relationship that must sit in the driver's seat. Next, in the Humanistic Stage, the lovers learn to bring their mind to the relationship, becoming more mindful of the importance of their lovemaking, more mindful of their obligation to be as fully loving as their circumstances permit all day long, and being mindful that sex represents something bigger than the lover's desire to please each other. Finally, the couple become truly soulful lovers, who understand, on an experiential level, that their physical love is a sign of the passion God himself longs to reveal to each of the lovers.

Throughout this section, we've discovered the treasure that is Holy Sex, and we've distinguished it from the fool's gold of eroticism. Further, I have attempted to illustrate that Holy Sex is superior because it requires the lovers to make a gift of their whole selves, not just the parts of themselves they are comfortable giving.

Having been introduced to the reality of Holy Sex, let's delve deeper into the mysteries of Infallible Loving.

PART TWO

The Five Great Powers of Holy Sex

S o far we've exposed some of the myths about the alleged "traditional Christian" views of sex and discovered the blueprint for becoming an Infallible Lover. Over the next five chapters, we explore the Five Powers that make Holy Sex a truly toe-curling, eye-popping, mind-blowing, deeply spiritual, and profoundly sacred experience.

What are the Five Powers possessed by Holy Sex? I thought you would never ask.

1. Holy Sex has the power to make the common holy.

2. Holy Sex has sacramental and redemptive power.

3. Holy Sex has the power to be a physical sign of God's passion for us.

4. Holy Sex has the power to unite.

5. Holy Sex has the power to create.

Readers should note carefully that the Five Powers do not apply in any meaningful way to recreational or promiscuous sex, which, as you have seen, is not sex at all, but merely eroticism. Though, superficially, eroticism has some things in common with Holy Sex, they are in fact completely different realities. Where Holy Sex draws transformative strength and supernatural significance from the Five Powers, eroticism is actually repelled by the Five Powers of Holy Sex. When the Five Powers of Holy Sex are activated by the graces of marriage, they go on a search-and-destroy mission, purging the couple's souls of eroticism while still enabling them to experience the fullness of a godly sensuality that is the root of both relational spirituality and authentic sexual pleasure.

The resistance the Five Powers of Holy Sex hold toward eroticism explains why so many people who have had such colorful premarital sex lives suddenly find they don't have the faintest clue of how to create a powerful marital sex life. The Five Powers reveal eroticism to be cheap, shallow, damaging, and ultimately as satisfying as a tall, cool glass of dirt.

Sex can be authentically human and, for that matter, authentically sexual only to the degree that it respects the Five Powers. The more a couple celebrates a love life that honors the holy, sacramental, symbolic, uniting, and creative power of sex, the more that couple will create a love life that is as soulful as it is inspiring and lifelong.

Quiz
TEST YOUR HOLY SEX QUOTIENT (HSQ)

The following quiz is intended to help you identify your Holy Sex Quotient, that is, your ability to fully tap into all Five Powers of Holy Sex and experience the fullness of what God intends married sex to be. The quiz will help you identify areas that you should pay attention to as you read the next few chapters on the Five Powers of Holy Sex. Write your score for each section of the quiz and then tally up all the scores to discover how much your sexual relationship takes advantage of the Five Powers. If you and your mate are reading the book together (which I recommend), both of you should take the quiz separately and discuss why you answered as you did.

The First Power:
Holy Sex Has the Power to Make the Common Holy

1. Holiness seems like something for saints and spiritual masters but not for me.

Disagree Totally	Disagree Somewhat	Neither Agree nor Disagree	Agree Somewhat	Agree Totally
5	4	3	2	1

2. The words "holiness" and "great sex" don't feel like they go together at all.

Disagree Totally	Disagree Somewhat	Neither Agree nor Disagree	Agree Somewhat	Agree Totally
5	4	3	2	1

3. Holy Sex sounds boring and "churchy."

Disagree Totally	Disagree Somewhat	Neither Agree nor Disagree	Agree Somewhat	Agree Totally
5	4	3	2	1

4. Being sensual is a requirement for being spiritual.

Disagree Totally	Disagree Somewhat	Neither Agree nor Disagree	Agree Somewhat	Agree Totally
1	2	3	4	5

5. Being spiritual doesn't necessarily require a commitment to change things about myself.

Disagree Totally	Disagree Somewhat	Neither Agree nor Disagree	Agree Somewhat	Agree Totally
5	4	3	2	1

First Power of Holy Sex score: _____ *out of a possible 25 points.*

The Second Power:
Holy Sex Has Sacramental and Redemptive Power

1. Becoming a great lover to my spouse plays a role in perfecting me as a person.

Disagree Totally	Disagree Somewhat	Neither Agree nor Disagree	Agree Somewhat	Agree Totally
1	2	3	4	5

2. Becoming a great lover to my spouse plays a role in helping me get to heaven.

Disagree Totally	Disagree Somewhat	Neither Agree nor Disagree	Agree Somewhat	Agree Totally
1	2	3	4	5

3. The sexual relationship between a husband and wife can tell us important things about God's relationship to humankind.

Disagree Totally	Disagree Somewhat	Neither Agree nor Disagree	Agree Somewhat	Agree Totally
1	2	3	4	5

4. Sex with my spouse is more like a chore than anything else.

Disagree Totally	Disagree Somewhat	Neither Agree nor Disagree	Agree Somewhat	Agree Totally
5	4	3	2	1

5. I am comfortable being vulnerable with others and able to inspire others to be vulnerable with me.

Disagree Totally	Disagree Somewhat	Neither Agree nor Disagree	Agree Somewhat	Agree Totally
1	2	3	4	5

Second Power of Holy Sex score: _____ *out of a possible 25 points.*

The Third Power:
Holy Sex Has the Power to Be a Physical Sign of God's Passion for Us

1. God uses physical things to make his love real for us.

Disagree Totally	Disagree Somewhat	Neither Agree nor Disagree	Agree Somewhat	Agree Totally
1	2	3	4	5

2. God uses the married couple's sexual relationship to show his love to both husband and wife.

Disagree Totally	Disagree Somewhat	Neither Agree nor Disagree	Agree Somewhat	Agree Totally
1	2	3	4	5

3. Loving each other "with God's love" sounds stifling and intimidating.

Disagree Totally	Disagree Somewhat	Neither Agree nor Disagree	Agree Somewhat	Agree Totally
5	4	3	2	1

4. If two people really love each other, great sex shouldn't take work; it should just happen.

Disagree Totally	Disagree Somewhat	Neither Agree nor Disagree	Agree Somewhat	Agree Totally
5	4	3	2	1

5. To be great, sex needs to be naughty.

Disagree Totally	Disagree Somewhat	Neither Agree nor Disagree	Agree Somewhat	Agree Totally
5	4	3	2	1

Third Power of Holy Sex score: _____ *out of a possible 25 points.*

The Fourth Power:
Holy Sex Has the Power to Unite

1. When a couple is in an ongoing sexual relationship, they increase their ability to influence each other's values, whatever they are.

Disagree Totally	Disagree Somewhat	Neither Agree nor Disagree	Agree Somewhat	Agree Totally
1	2	3	4	5

2. When two people have sex, a bond is formed only if they love each other.

Disagree Totally	Disagree Somewhat	Neither Agree nor Disagree	Agree Somewhat	Agree Totally
5	4	3	2	1

3. Sex can change people for better or worse.

Disagree Totally	Disagree Somewhat	Neither Agree nor Disagree	Agree Somewhat	Agree Totally
1	2	3	4	5

4. Contraception (e.g., barrier methods such as condoms; the Pill) does not impact the ability of sex to bond lovers together.

Disagree Totally	Disagree Somewhat	Neither Agree nor Disagree	Agree Somewhat	Agree Totally
5	4	3	2	1

5. Healthy sex in marriage unites the husband and wife to each other and God.

Disagree Totally	Disagree Somewhat	Neither Agree nor Disagree	Agree Somewhat	Agree Totally
1	2	3	4	5

Fourth Power of Holy Sex score: _____ *out of a possible 25 points.*

The Fifth Power:
Holy Sex Has the Power to Create

1. For Catholics, the desire to have babies is the only legitimate reason to have sex.

Disagree Totally	Disagree Somewhat	Neither Agree nor Disagree	Agree Somewhat	Agree Totally
5	4	3	2	1

2. It's only natural that marital intimacy decreases after children are born.

Disagree Totally	Disagree Somewhat	Neither Agree nor Disagree	Agree Somewhat	Agree Totally
5	4	3	2	1

3. There is no such thing as a great sex life after kids.

Disagree Totally	Disagree Somewhat	Neither Agree nor Disagree	Agree Somewhat	Agree Totally
5	4	3	2	1

4. Openness to life and openness to conception are the same exact thing.

Disagree Totally	Disagree Somewhat	Neither Agree nor Disagree	Agree Somewhat	Agree Totally
5	4	3	2	1

5. The unwillingness to have children (or to have more children) has no effect on a couple's sexual intimacy.

Disagree Totally	Disagree Somewhat	Neither Agree nor Disagree	Agree Somewhat	Agree Totally
5	4	3	2	1

Fifth Power of Holy Sex score: _____ *out of a possible 25 points.*

SCORING
WHAT'S YOUR HSQ?

Total your points for all five sections: _____ *out of a possible 125 points.*

- ◆ Which of the Five Powers did you score the highest in?
- ◆ Which of the Five Powers did you score the lowest in?

A score of...

112–125: Outstanding! Much about Holy Sex comes naturally to you. Your sexual relationship is most likely highly satisfying and representative of the love you share all day long. You are truly soulful, passionate lovers.

98–111: Your sexual relationship is definitely above average. You are aware of the spiritual dimensions of your sexuality, and you want to be mindful of those dimensions in lovemaking. You may have occasional disagreements about sex, but overall you usually handle them well and are confident in your love for each other. Even so, you may sometimes struggle with what integrating your spirituality and sexuality really means — practically speaking. Pay attention to new ways to practice the Five Powers of Holy Sex so that you can more completely experience what you know sex can be.

76–97: Your sexual relationship just isn't all it could be. Miscommunication around sexual issues, unequal desire, and the tendency to take the sexual relationship for granted are all common, but potentially serious, difficulties for couples who score in this range. You have a lot of strengths to work with, but you probably haven't spent a lot of time thinking about what your sexual relationship says about you as a total person or about the overall health of your marital relationship. Use the areas you scored strongest in as the foundation for creating deeper intimacy. You may also wish to enlist the help of faithful counseling to overcome faulty beliefs or bad relationship habits that are negatively affecting your sexual relationship. For additional information, contact the Pastoral Solutions Institute (*www.exceptionalmarriages.com*).

25–75: You are most likely dissatisfied with your sexual relationship.
You may also be experiencing resentment or anger related to your sex
life and relationship in general. The good news is that you have the opportunity to start fresh. Pay attention to how different Holy Sex is to
what you've been experiencing and complete the exercises in this book
to remodel your sexual lives. For additional support, contact the Pastoral
Solutions Institute (see above).

You're in This Together

One word of caution: If both you and your mate have taken the quiz, it's
possible that one spouse might record a high overall score while his or her
mate records a very low overall score. If this happens, this doesn't mean
that one person is a great Infallible Lover while the other is a stick-in-
the-mud. It means that the high scorer probably thinks a little too well
of himself or herself! Holy Sex is definitely a cooperative enterprise. One
principle of Infallible Loving is that the sexual relationship is only as good
as both partners think it is. If there's a wide disparity between your scores,
consider what that may mean about your ability to truly understand and
attend to each other.

Regardless of your score, as you review the next few chapters, explore
the ways you can more completely integrate the spiritual dimensions of
your sexual relationship and experience the fullness of what God intends
your intimate lives to be.

5   SEX MAKES US HOLY

Undeniably, in heaven we shall see, we shall love, and we shall praise. Our vision will never fail, our love will never end, and our praise will never fall silent. Love sings now; then, too, it is a love that will sing. But now it is a yearning love that sings; then it will be an enjoying love.
— St. Augustine, *Sermon 254,6*

To be an Infallible Lover, the first thing you must recognize is that sex is and must always be *holy*. It must make you holy. It must make your beloved holy. It must lead you to Him who is holy.

Although we addressed this question briefly in our argument against the McGillicuddy-ites, the first of the Five Powers — the power of sex to make the common holy — is so life-changing that it is worth a closer look. Remember, when Catholics say that sex is holy, we don't mean it in the "touch it and die" sense of the Jansenists, but in the incarnational, divinized-nature sense of holiness. Sex is holy because Jesus' incarnation and our participation in the life of grace through baptism makes *us* holy (see CCC no. 460). Therefore, sex becomes the most intimate way one divinized human person can share himself or herself completely with another divinized human person.

WHAT DOES HOLY MEAN?

What does it mean to be holy? Perhaps it means that you have the power to glow in the dark? Or fly? Or be in two places at the same time? Or read souls or minds or hearts? While all those paranormal powers would be really cool to have (and some saints have had them), none of them are specifically indicators of holiness. After all, as Scripture notes, signs and wonders can be of divine or diabolical origin. Rather than defining holiness in terms of superpowers, St. Thomas Aquinas argued that holiness is the virtue that places a person, a thing, or an action in the service of God. *If something is holy, it simply means that it has been set apart for a divine purpose.* Water set aside for baptism becomes holy water. Bread and wine set aside for the purpose of nourishing our souls become Holy Communion. Someone whose life becomes an example of what it means to set oneself aside to do God's will — Mother Teresa or St. Francis of Assisi, for instance — is a saint, a holy man or woman.

Holiness takes common things and makes them special and more significant than they could ever be on their own. The act of setting something aside for a divine purpose, whether a thing, an activity, or a person, transforms it in some way that goes beyond our senses or the mere significance assigned to it by believers. Even most nonbelievers feel a sense of awe and respect when they enter a church. Even most nonbelievers would think twice before using the chalice that holds the Precious Blood as a spittoon. Even most nonbelievers were inspired merely to be in the presence of Mother Teresa or Pope John Paul II. But why? A church is just a building. A chalice is just a cup. Mother Teresa and Pope John Paul II were just folks. Except, virtually everyone knows they are not. The act of setting aside something, or oneself, for a divine purpose doesn't just make it more significant for believers; it changes the nature of the thing. It transforms the person or object in a way that defies description but is tangible nonetheless. As St. Thomas Aquinas's great Eucharistic hymn so beautifully states, "Praestet fides supplementum, sensuum defectui." Even when our senses fail us, our souls know that some things are more than they seem.

The same is true about Holy Sex. Sex, in and of itself, is really nothing special. In fact, it is one of the most common facts of nature. Birds do it. Bees do it. Even *un*educated fleas do it. If you have the intelligence of a fruit fly, you can have sex. Two teenagers in the back seat of a car or two strangers in the night or ten people at a sex club are not really doing anything that your average rabbit or lab rat couldn't manage competently enough.

The Five Great Powers of Holy Sex

But Holy Sex is a different story entirely. Only humans can set sex aside to serve the divine purpose for which it was created. Holy Sex makes the common holy. It transforms the lovers and the love they share into a powerful, mystical reality that not only bonds the couple together, but images God's love for his creation. Holy Sex makes God's own love for the couple discernible to the senses. It challenges the couple to reach for the heights of generosity and compels them to celebrate the generative impulse through both childbearing and other loving acts. Holy Sex takes something that is common and ordains it to do things it shouldn't be able to do on its own, but can, because it has been infused with the grace of marriage. Discovering and celebrating the divine purpose of sex transforms the very nature of sex itself. It becomes Holy Sex.

Holy Sex is *godly* sex in the sense that it enables you to love with the power of God. Of course, depending on your idea of who God is and how God relates to us, the idea of godly sex may not exactly rev your engines. But it should. Remember, more than anything, "God is a lover." As the epigraphs that begin each chapter attest, this theme echoes throughout Christian mystical spirituality. Thomas à Kempis's great spiritual classic, *The Imitation of Christ*, refers to God as the "Divine Lover." St. Catherine of Siena goes old Tommy one better and refers to God as her "Mad Lover." One could hardly find a more beautiful representation of the role of God as ravisher of his beloved than the famous statue by Bernini, *The Transverberation of St. Teresa of Avila*, which illustrates the passionate power of an ecstatic, heavenly union between divine bridegroom and beloved bride.

Christian tradition makes it pretty clear that God is no slouch as a lover either. Saints who experienced theophanies (powerful, personal, and very real encounters with the divine presence of God) didn't refer to the experience as "being in ecstasy" for nothing.

Bringing this concept of theophany a little closer to home, the Eucharist, the "source and summit" of the Catholic faith (see CCC no. 1324), is chock-full of powerful imagery of God as our Divine Lover. The Eucharist is nothing if not an epic love story culminating in one of the most

98

beautiful love scenes of human history. Let's see if I can't set the scene for you.

Once upon a time, there was a bride held captive by a demonic evil prince. To ransom his beloved (us, his Church), Christ, the Divine Lover, suffered, died, and rose again for the sake of a love so powerful that neither death nor the gates of hell could prevail against it. Having won his prize, the salvation of his bride, he now gives himself to us completely — body, soul, and divinity — through the Most Holy Sacrament of the Altar. We draw him close. He enters us. His flesh becomes one with our flesh. His blood courses through our veins. Fearful and eager at once to be completely vulnerable to him, we fall prey to his all-consuming love. Inspired by his passion, nourished by his loving embrace, and propelled by the power of his Holy Spirit alive within us, we enter the world again, refreshed and renewed — ready to do the great work of bringing new children to him through the waters of baptism.

Pope John Paul II was especially keen on this image of the Eucharist. In his book *Love and Responsibility*, Karol Wojtyla (a.k.a. "The man who would be pope") argues that the Eucharist is the source of the sacrament of matrimony. Dr. Mary Rousseau wrote a wonderful essay entitled "Eucharist and Gender," beautifully summarizing this powerful concept:

Pope John Paul II rightly refers to the Eucharist as the source of the Sacrament of Matrimony, which in turn is the source of families and, through families, of the Civilization of Love. There is, indeed, a most intimate connection between the Sacrament of Matrimony and the Eucharist. Jesus' love is the love of a Bridegroom for his Bride. The Mass itself, as his continuing free acceptance of his death, is a marital act. Indeed, it is the marital act of all marital acts. Unlike other references to the relation of Christ to the Church, such as Shepherd to sheep, King to subjects, and so on, the Bridegroom-to-Bride reference is primary and non-figurative. It is not a metaphor, but a literal statement that Jesus' love for us is marital. It is, of course, not sexual, not reproductive in a physical way. But the fact of divine marital love tells us something about the core essence of human marital love. Like our Lord's love for us, human marital love must be completely self-giving, free of any self-seeking — it must be unconditional, gratuitous, faithful, permanent, and given to no rivals. Matrimony, then, as a sacrament, is a causal symbol of that primary, divine marital love. And human marital love is sexual. In fact, sexual intercourse is integral to the sacramental symbol.

Clearly, for the Catholic Christian, who thinks of sexual love as the most appropriate image for the union between the divine bridegroom and his beloved, there is nothing shameful or second-rate about Holy Sex. For the Christian, sex is a sign and a foreshadowing of the union that God longs to celebrate with each and every one of us. Of course, as Mary Rousseau notes, divine love is not sexual in a reproductive sense, but it is certainly marital, unitive, and passionate. Sex is so important to the Christian that Pope John Paul II referred to marriage — the sacrament of sex (it ain't the sacrament of doing dishes together) — as "the primordial sacrament." Just like the so-called "primordial soup" contained and fore-shadowed all life on the planet, marriage, given by God to Adam and Eve in the beginning of time, contained and foreshadowed our life in grace and revealed God's plan to unite all of humankind to each other and to himself. The sacraments are entirely about achieving union with God. In Ephesians 5:32, St. Paul argues that marriage is a "great mystery" revealing the union between the Divine Lover and his beloved. Marriage is the first sacrament, given by God to our first parents in the garden. When God in-structed Adam and Eve to "go forth and multiply," he wasn't giving them math homework. He had much more up the giant sleeve of his big, puffy white robe. When God gave marriage to Adam and Eve, he was instituting a relationship that both signified and actualized the nuptial unity between man, woman, and himself. After the Fall, when the relationship between man, woman, and God was torn apart, God sought to restore that original unity. He sent Christ, his Son, the bridegroom who, by his incarnation, passion, death, and resurrection — and by means of the sacraments he instituted to continue his ministry into the present day — reclaims his bride and empowers us to strive for the union we enjoyed with God at the dawn of creation.

In short, God longs to unite with us and share with us the joy he experiences in that union. In the words of the *Encyclopedia of Catholic Doctrine,* "God created the whole universe so that new beings might be able to share in the unimaginable richness of his being. He created human beings to share eternal bliss with him." Nowhere is this more true than in the human sexual relationship, which is truly an image of God's love affair with creation. Indeed, to experience Holy Sex is to experience the cataclysmic eruption of love that was the cosmological orgasm physicists refer to as "the Big Bang," through which the entire universe was created and from which the entire universe continues to reel even today. Who wouldn't give his eyeteeth for a night like that with his beloved?

And that's why the First Power of Holy Sex, the power to make the common holy, is not an intimidating or passion-killing notion, but rather a life-giving, explosive, transformative reality. Imagine the shock you'd get if you stuck your tongue on a lightning rod in the middle of an electrical storm. As powerful as that would be, it's got nothing on Holy Sex. When a couple celebrates Holy Sex, they're tapping into the cataclysmic, divine spark of passionate love that created the universe, overcame the gates of hell, destroyed death, and culminated in the creation of you. As St. Paul notes in Ephesians 5, Holy Sex bears witness to the most powerful love in the universe. Clearly, we're not talking about kids' stuff.

SENSUAL AND SPIRITUAL

One problem that many people have with trying to wrap their heads around the idea that sex is holy is that many of us have a decidedly in-complete view of what it means to be spiritual. If you turn on your favorite women's daytime talk program or go to the "spirituality" section of your local bookstore, you'll walk away with the idea that the path to spiritual enlightenment involves burning scented candles, getting massages, and taking long hot baths while listening to some bald guy play elevator music on a pan flute. If this is your image of what it means to be "spiritual," well, you're only half right.

Surprised that I'm giving such a person even a 50 percent grade on their spirituality quiz? Don't be. The part that such a person gets right is that spirituality does involve the senses (though I personally discourage the whole pan flute thing). In fact, sensuality is a first step in spirituality. That's why Catholic churches and Catholic liturgy are so, well, *sensual*. Throughout history — and even to this day — many Protestants have been absolutely scandalized by all the "smells and bells" Catholics use in worship. Let the cotton-bloomer-ed, blue-haired Puritan church ladies shriek. *Benedicamus Domino!* Catholics are proud of our sensual roots.

Of course, thanks to the National Association of Conventional Wisdom on All Things Catholic and their powerful friends in Big Media, the Catholic Church gets a lot of flack for being "anti-pleasure," but nothing could be further from the truth. When it comes to sex, the Church is very pro-pleasure. In fact, there are some Catholic theologians (such as Pope John Paul II) who have argued that a husband has an *obligation* to see that his wife achieves orgasm. Think on this for a moment. Rather than suggesting that pleasure is bad, official Church teaching insists that both husband and wife have a *right* to expect the heights of pleasure from their sexual relationship. Furthermore, in *Love and Responsibility*, Karol Wojtyla argued that a husband and wife should strive to achieve orgasm simultaneously because the simultaneous orgasm is the most powerful sign whereby a woman and man give themselves to each other totally. That's right: Catholics "hate" sex and pleasure so much that an archbishop-who-would-be-pope took time out of his busy schedule to encourage married couples to pursue the heights of sexual pleasure.

No doubt this might seem a bit much for many of you. I recall an article in *Commonweal* that contained the following satirical look at Pope John Paul II's theologizing about sex:

> I learned that the goal of sex within marriage is "perfect self-donation" and
> how "true attraction desires the other's good through the gift of myself."

A line, I confess, that I have on occasion used myself. But when I came upon [Catholic theologian George] Weigel's pithy summary of John Paul's theology of sex, I felt compelled to call my wife back into the room. Marriage, after all, is a "school where we become fitted . . . to make a complete gift of self to the other." I could not, in good conscience, spare her this.

"Darling," I said, my eyes alight in hopeful expectation, "would you say that our sex life 'is an icon of the interior life of God'?"

Honesty compels me to report that a moment of awkward silence followed. My wife then gave me what I can only describe as a pitying look.

"Just let me explain . . . ," I protested.

She smiled patronizingly, patted me on the shoulder in the spirit of "mutual self-giving," and headed out of the room. "I don't understand how you can read that stuff," she said, shaking her head.

People like this writer (i.e., most people) don't get what Catholics really think about sex because they think of themselves as animals, *but the Church thinks of humans as gods.* As the *Catechism of the Catholic Church* no. 460 states, "The son of God became man so that we might become God." The world tells you to think about sex as animals do. But *the Church wants you to make love like a god.* Infallible Lovers know this, and strive to rise to the happy challenge.

Clearly, the Church doesn't have a problem with pleasure, so what's the problem? While the Church recognizes and celebrates the greatness of pleasure, the Church recognizes that respecting the dignity of your lover and yourself is an even greater pleasure. And giving pleasure to one another in a manner that is also deeply respectful and authentically loving is the greatest pleasure of all. That's why Catholics discourage inferior expressions of sex and call them sins, because they are *less good* than what God really wants you to have: the *sex life of a god.* Or as Pope Benedict XVI writes, the Church would have you celebrate "true *eros* [which] tends to rise 'in ecstasy' toward the Divine, to lead us beyond ourselves."

As Pope Benedict's quotation asserts, sensuality can't be where the journey ends. In his book *Integrating Spirituality and Counseling,* psychotherapist

Dr. E. Hinterkopf defines spiritual experience as "a subtle, bodily feeling with vague meanings that brings new clearer meanings involving a transcendent growth process."

In other words spirituality involves two components: a sensual *call* followed by an intentional growth *response*. Sensuality is what is referred to in the first part of his definition: "a subtle, bodily feeling with vague meaning." The growth response is contained in the second part of Hinterkopf's definition: that which "brings new clearer meanings involving a transcendent growth process." Both components — sensuality and transcendent growth response — are necessary for an experience to be truly "spiritual."

I'm using a secular definition of spirituality specifically because I want to demonstrate that I'm not being religiously triumphalistic. Though many people experience spirituality differently, there is agreement between religious people and the secular professions who study spiritual experience about exactly what authentic spirituality entails. Even so, a lot of people with a specifically secular mind-set can become genuinely irritated when confronted with the fact that sensuality is only one part of authentic spirituality. I remember counseling one couple in which the wife was religiously devout but her husband was not. Although both had their problems, the husband was especially narcissistic. He didn't believe in extending himself for anyone under any circumstances if he didn't feel like it. He lived a life dedicated to his feelings and pursuing new sensual experiences. When the topic turned to their religious differences, the husband asserted that he was "spiritual" and that he didn't need religion, because he experienced God in nature, in music, or in certain reportedly incredible sexual experiences he'd had with past girlfriends. I challenged him about his concept of spirituality, especially on the last example. I told him that these experiences were deeply sensual, but that they lacked an important component for being truly spiritual. Before I had a chance to explain myself, he looked at me and said, "Buddy, you don't know my old girlfriend. She could. . . ." He trailed off and then said, "Just trust me. It was plenty spiritual." This guy, like so many people, was missing the point.

If I listen to a stirring symphony, watch a beautiful sunrise, eat a wonderful meal, or have a passionate night of lovemaking with my wife, I'm having a sensual experience. But as beautiful as that can be, so far, it's merely a sensual experience and not, as many people think, a spiritual one. If, however, going to the symphony makes me want to praise God for all of his glory, or viewing the sunrise gives me a sense of gratitude for nature that motivates me to honor God's creation by spending the next weekend picking up litter in my neighborhood, or if making love with my wife makes me want to dedicate my entire life to loving her as God himself loves her, *then* my sensual experience motivates an expansive response — part of a transcendent growth process — and that experience has been truly spiritual. God calls to me through my senses, and if I respond, a brilliant spark arcs across the distance between God and the human person, creating the bridge we experience as spirituality.

In his book *Surprised by Joy,* C. S. Lewis tells the story of his conversion. He describes in some detail his enjoyment of certain things — literature, nature, and the like. At some point, he begins to realize, almost all at once, that these things he enjoys point to something else entirely. They point to Joy, God, himself.

> *This discovery flashed a new light back on my whole life. I saw that all my waitings and watchings for Joy ... had been a futile attempt to contemplate the enjoyed. All that such watching and waiting ever could find would be ... an image. I know now that they were merely the mental track left by the passage of Joy — not the wave but the wave's imprint on the sand. The inherent dialectic of desire itself had already shown me this; for all images and sensations, if idolatrously mistaken for Joy itself, soon honestly confessed themselves inadequate. All said, in the last resort, "It is not I. I am only the reminder. Look! Look! What do I remind you of?"*

Holy Sex, because it is intimately connected to God, the source of all joy and love, has the power to make the common holy because, when we approach it with the eyes of our soul wide open, we recognize that the sensual experience of lovemaking points to something bigger, something greater, something even more amazing. It points to the joy we will experience when, at long last, we fling ourselves into the arms of our Divine Lover, loving and being loved so completely that we will spend all of eternity crying out in heavenly union with all the angels and saints, "Holy! Holy! Holy!"

6 SEX IS SACRAMENTAL

Christian Marriage, like the other sacraments, whose purpose is to sanctify God's people, to build up the body of Christ, and finally, to give worship to God, is in itself a liturgical action glorifying God in Jesus Christ and in the Church. By celebrating it, Christian spouses profess their gratitude to God for the sublime gift bestowed on them of being able to live in their married and family lives the very love of God for people and that of the Lord Jesus Christ for the Church, his bride.
— Pope John Paul II, *Familiaris Consortio*

A re you sitting down? This next point is a bit of a shock to the system for some people. You might want to make sure you have something soft and cushy to faint on just in case you're overcome. Ready? Okay. In addition to having the power to make the common holy, Holy Sex has the power to be *sacramental* and *redemptive*.

Most people have one of three reactions to this.

1. They may laugh out loud at the ridiculousness of it.

2. They may be appalled and offended.

3. They may stare at you, nodding politely until you stop speaking and then ask you to pass the salt.

While all of these reactions are understandable, none of them is really appropriate. Let's take a closer look at the sacramental and redemptive power of sex and see if we can't make a little more sense of this idea.

First of all, what does the word "sacrament" mean? Traditionally, Catholics define sacrament as an outward sign that was instituted by Christ to give us grace. But grace to do what? To be united to God through Christ and to be perfected in love (Matt. 5:48). So just to be sure we're clear, when the Church says that marriage is a sacrament, the Church is saying that the sexual relationship between man and woman has been given to us by God as a means of signifying and facilitating a union between the man, woman, and God himself and to help the husband and wife be perfected in love.

That's a powerful statement. Unfortunately, it's completely antithetical to most people's experience of sex. Again, most people don't know a thing about Holy Sex; they know only about eroticism. And as I've already mentioned in my brief introduction to Part Two, the Five Powers of Holy Sex do not apply to eroticism.

Can this idea of the sacramental nature of sexuality — that is, that sex at its core is a sign instituted by God to give grace — be sustained in Christian tradition? The notion is certainly biblical. As we've noted in our discussion of the First Power of Holy Sex, God instituted marriage at the dawn of creation when he gave Eve to Adam and told them to "go forth and multiply." Jesus, when responding to his disciples regarding their questions about divorce, skips right over Mosaic tradition and asks his followers to remember what God intended for marriage "from the beginning" (Matt. 19:8). By doing so, Jesus clearly indicates that God, not man-made tradition, is the real author of marriage (therefore meeting the first criterion necessary to be considered a sacrament) and that God had a specific plan in mind when he created it.

And what could that plan be? We find one part of that answer in Ephesians (5:21 and following) when St. Paul reminds us marriage is a sign of the union between Christ and the Church. I'm not sure what most people think when they read this passage, but Catholic tradition, and especially the work of Pope John Paul II, asserts that St. Paul is referring to the fact that the sexual union between man and woman itself says something about the nature of God's union with us. In particular, St. Paul is telling us that the nature of God's love is nuptial — not sexual in the reproductive sense, but nuptial. God's union with us can be best understood by humans as the intimate union between a husband and wife in which God pours his love into creation and creation receives that love leading to the bursting forth of greater life in the spirit.

A MARRIAGE MADE FOR HEAVEN

In John 2:1–11, Jesus dignifies marriage by making it the occasion of his first miracle. Most people think this was just a chance occurrence. Perhaps if Jesus had been at a birthday party, he would have been asked to make more cake out of confetti. What if he'd been invited to a kegger at the University of Nazareth? Would he make sure the party was never tapped out? Nonsense.

The Church asserts that this moment was ordained for Christ to reveal himself because Christ's union with humankind is a nuptial union. There is nothing accidental about Jesus' choices. Jesus, at the insistence of his Blessed Mother — who knew a thing or two about union with God — chose the moment of the wedding feast of Cana to reveal himself as the world's bridegroom. In his document on the rosary (*Rosarium Virginis Mariae*), Pope John Paul II proposed the addition of five new mysteries, the Luminous Mysteries or Mysteries of Light, of which the miracle at Cana is one. Pope John Paul II explained that the Mysteries of Light were meant to help the faithful contemplate the "revelation of the Kingdom now present in the very person of Jesus." In particular, the miracle at Cana reveals the nuptial nature of the Kingdom Jesus came to make present to humankind.

All of this is to say that when a man and woman celebrate, not just any old sex, but Holy Sex in the context of marriage, there is much more going on than meets the eye. In particular, Holy Sex both signifies and effects the union of the man, woman, and God and helps perfect both the husband and wife in love.

Now, let's get back to the bedroom.

Catholics believe that every time married people make love they are celebrating the sacrament of matrimony. The Church teaches that every time a Christian married couple makes love, they are physically restating their marriage vows and recommitting themselves to all the promises they made at the altar. Every time a Christian married couple makes love, they promise — using a language that can only be spoken by one ensouled body to another — to love, honor, and cherish, in good times and bad, sickness and health, wealth and poverty, all the days of their life, till death do them part. So many couples look forward to their twenty-fifth anniversary when they, by popular tradition, get to stand up and renew their vows, but no married couple has to wait that long. You can renew your vows tonight — or right now — if your mate is available.

The notion that sex can be sacramental, and even redemptive, is a completely shocking statement, though, and completely absurd to anyone whose sexual experience and education has been primarily rooted in eroticism instead of Holy Sex. Think about it. The sacraments are primarily concerned with sanctification — which is all about attaining heaven. But what could sex possibly have to do with eternal life? We will return to this theme again and again and explore this idea in much greater detail throughout the book, but here I want to emphasize the following:

When I die, I'm going to stand before the Almighty and all his glory — in all *my* glory. Every blemish, wrinkle, crease, and bump of a physical, emotional, and spiritual being will be — for all eternity — exposed to his penetrating gaze, vulnerable to his pervasive touch. Under such circumstances, in order for me to experience anything other than the sheer terror of hell, I must be able to stand confidently in the presence of that gaze, like Adam and Eve while they still enjoyed their original innocence. What better way for me to prepare myself for this awesome encounter with my Divine Lover than to challenge whatever vulnerability or shame I feel when my wife gazes upon me in my nakedness and makes love with me — and vice versa? It is this unique power of Infallible Sex to challenge unhealthy shame and expand our capacity for authentic vulnerability at the deepest level of our personhood that, in addition to its power to unite and create, makes sex a sanctifying, purifying reality.

The notion that love could be terrifying may strike some readers as odd at first glance, but it's not odd at all. What comes less naturally to us fallen, broken, wounded human beings than loving and being loved? Yet, that's exactly what we're destined to spend eternity doing. To be unable to do this is to be in hell. St. Augustine was once famously asked what God does to the souls in hell. He responded, "He loves them."

In a sense, hell is little more than the flames of God's love licking at the hearts of those who cannot melt. Let me offer a comparison that might make a little more sense. My clinical practice is filled with men and women so wounded and broken that it hurts to be loved. For some, the pain is so great they would rather reject love altogether than be forced to expose their hearts and souls to someone — even a gentle, caring someone — and have nowhere to hide. Here is how one female client, Kara, described her difficulties relating to the first healthy relationship of her adulthood.

All my life, nobody ever really loved me unless they could get something out of me. Now that I've found a really good man, I don't know what to do with him. I keep waiting for the axe to fall. He's patient, loving, sensitive. He's never done anything to make me doubt him, but I can't let my guard down. I can't accept the fact that he loves me. I want to shake him and say, "What's wrong with you! Can't you see how f***ed up I am!" I want to push him away. I hate myself for not believing him. I hate putting him through this. Sometimes I hate him for loving me.

While I hope most readers won't find themselves this alienated from love, all of us struggle with the awkwardness and fear of exposing the best and the worst parts of ourselves to our lover, no matter how caring and gentle he or she is. Now imagine this fear on an exponential scale, an eternal scale. Wounded by sin, unaccustomed to either giving or receiving real love, we are suddenly thrust into the presence of Real Love himself. All at once, we find ourselves forced by the circumstances of eternity to actively participate in the most intense, in-your-face, passionate, authentic love relationship we've ever encountered. I can't think of anything more terrifying, especially for those who have spent a lifetime guarding their hearts under lock and key. And yet, in the Infallible Lovemaking that occurs between man and woman in the sacrament of matrimony, husband and wife challenge this basic shame, fear, and self-doubt. Together, with God's grace, the man and woman create the safety that makes healthy vulnerability possible: the vulnerability that is required if one wishes to give and receive real love.

SARA AND ANGELO'S STORY

Sara and Angelo have been married thirty years and have five children. Sara was a virgin when she married Angelo. Her sexual education consisted of her parents telling her that bad things happen to girls who don't wait to have sex until marriage, and that if she ever decided to ignore their advice and she got pregnant, she'd be "out on her ass." She developed a suspicious, cautious attitude toward sex that continued well into her married years. As Sara puts it, "I just couldn't understand how one minute I shouldn't do this thing that was really bad for you, and then the next minute, because we went to church and the priest said some words, everything was suddenly okay. What made sex good all of a sudden?"

By contrast, Angelo had been sexually active prior to marriage with a handful of partners. His experiences ranged from a few one-night stands in college to a longer-term relationship with a young woman he lived with for about six months. Rather than being suspicious of sex, Angelo's experience taught him to treat sex as an entitlement. In the early years of his marriage to Sara, he would act personally offended when Sara would indicate that she didn't want to be intimate on a particular evening, and he would regularly complain that she wasn't generous enough.

Like many couples, Sara and Angelo had a lot to learn about how to tap into the sacramental and redemptive power of Holy Sex. As Sara puts it, "In the beginning, neither of us really knew what sex was supposed to be in marriage. I didn't know what to do with it. Nobody ever taught me. And Angelo thought marriage was some kind of fun pass to fantasyland."

Angelo agreed. "I hate to admit it, but she's right. At first, I thought about sex in terms of what it did for me. I used to tell myself I was trying to love Sara and she was just being mean and frigid by not doing it as often as I wanted, but really I wasn't caring what she needed from me. I just wanted what I wanted."

The turning point for them came after their second child. Sara was feeling overwhelmed with the responsibilities of having two children under four and was still doing part-time work at the city library. Angelo volunteered to take more responsibility for the house and meals to help lighten her load. Moreover, they went on a Marriage Encounter weekend that got them talking on a new level.

"Between Angelo's extra help and the conversations we had after that weekend," says Sara, "Angelo and I started to understand each other better. Mostly it was his volunteering to help more that showed me he really did love me. That I wasn't just there to service his sexual needs."

Angelo said that his increased service taught him something too. "When I started looking for ways I could be more helpful, for some reason I started to think more about sex in terms of service. I mean, that sex was supposed to be one of the things I could do to take care of Sara, but she experienced lovemaking as me taking something from her. It dawned on me that maybe the reason for that wasn't so much that she was uptight, but that I was approaching the whole thing too selfishly. I didn't realize it then, but looking back, I think God whacked me on the head and said, 'Hey, Ange, you moron, I don't act like a selfish jerk to you! What you doin' treatin' this lady I gave you like that?'"

"To be fair," adds Sara, "I was too uptight. I was kind of ashamed of my body and sex in general. But when he backed off and focused on just loving me instead of demanding sex like it was some kind of husbandly right, I could relax and start to love him better. I could feel that there was something more going on between us. It wasn't just Angelo loving me. It was like we were sharing something p urer that made me want to be more vulnerable, more adventurous, more open."

Sara and Angelo report that after many years of serving one another and learning to talk openly about what they needed from each other, their sexual relationship has not only become truly dynamic and soulful, but it's also been the catalyst for changes in who they are as people.

Sara explains, "I didn't know anything about this when I first got married. I thought sex was just sex. But working on our sexual relationship made us really look at how to be better people. Back then, we were both immature and selfish in our own ways. Now, we have become more real. I mean, more generous, more selfless."

Sara and Angelo's willingness to struggle with the fallen sexual attitudes of their early years challenged them to become more mature, selfless, generous lovers in and out of the bedroom. The love they shared over the years — and continue to share — illustrates the power of sex to perfect the husband and wife in love and enable each other to share a love that is rooted in God's passion rather than their own.

TAKING SEX FOR GRANTED

The case of Sara and Angelo illustrates the power of Holy Sex to redeem the selfish parts of ourselves and prepare us to be better examples of God's love for each other. But there is yet another benefit that the Second Power of Holy Sex, the power to be sacramental and redemptive, brings to marriage, namely, because it stops a couple from ever forgetting the transformative power and spiritual significance of their sexual love, it prevents them from taking their sexual relationship for granted.

Because lovemaking is a reenactment of all the joys and promises of the wedding day, Christian married couples must never take their sexuality for granted. Let's think again about an example we used earlier. Did you take your wedding day for granted? Did you decide not to show up for the ceremony just because you were tired or stressed? (I was both, but it didn't stop me, nor, thank God, my wife, from coming down the aisle.) Did you say to the pastor witnessing your ceremony, "Can we move this along, Father? We've got a lot to do tomorrow, and I'd like to turn in early tonight." Of course you didn't. You'd been looking forward to your wedding day your whole life and planning it since the Paleozoic Era. Tired as you may have been, you drew strength from your wedding day. You hung on every word, sign, and gesture.

Every married couple who understands the truth of Christian sexuality views their ongoing sexual relationship in the same way.

In today's work-centered (as opposed to love-centered) world, one of the fastest growing sexual disorders is Hypoactive Sexual Desire Disorder (HSDD). One of the chief causes of HSDD, according to research, is that most couples place their sex lives at the bottom of their priority list. They have so many other things to do that by the time they fall into bed at night, they barely have enough strength to acknowledge that there is someone else in the room, much less make love. As secular marriage therapist Michelle Wiener-Davis writes in her book *The Sex-Starved Marriage:*

> *There's no question about it. Our lives are hectic. . . . Stress takes a toll on our bodies. It makes sleep hard to come by. Your energy level takes a dip. It weakens your immune system and you often become ill. Your body often starts hurting as if to say, "Help, slow down!" You are on overload. You feel frazzled much of the time. Nothing seems like fun anymore, not even sex. When sex starts feeling like a chore, it often gets moved to the last chore on your to-do list.*

But Christian married couples who understand their lovemaking as a restatement of their wedding vows rarely, if ever, fall prey to HSDD. How could they? Sure, they get stressed like everyone else, but just like a newlywed couple's wedding day is energizing and life-giving to the couple who should otherwise be dead on their feet from months of fighting with caterers, in-laws, musicians, and assorted other wedding nuisances, the properly disposed Christian couple experiences each private "wedding celebration" of lovemaking as a beautiful, life-giving, energizing, desirable event. No matter how tired they are, they want to fall into the comforting arms of their best friend and lover. Such a couple can't wait to walk down the aisle to their bedroom (or any other room, for that matter) and renew their vows on the altar that is their marriage bed (or sofa, or dining room table, or stairway, or . . .). To such a couple, sex is not "just one more thing on the to-do list": it is the fountain from which they drink to grow in love and celebrate the partnership that daily helps them become who God created them to be. Christian married couples with a deeply spiritual sexuality spend as much time and energy nurturing, planning, and rejoicing in the *private, physical* celebrations of their wedding day as they did nurturing, planning, and rejoicing in the *public* celebration of their first wedding day. They do this because they realize how beautiful and how essential lovemaking is to the core of their married vocation.

In sum, the Second Power of Holy Sex, the power to make marital love-making a redemptive and sacramental reality, yields four major benefits. It challenges a husband and wife to overcome the shame and vulnerability they experience in the presence of Real Love. It challenges the husband and wife to love one another with the selfless love God gives them, rather than just with their own fallen concepts of love. It allows a husband and wife to experience a physical sign of the nuptial reality of God's relation-ship with each of us. And finally, it keeps the sexual relationship fresh by imbuing it with a significance that goes well beyond momentary pleasure or recreation.

7 SEX IS A SIGN OF GOD'S LOVE

O pure and holy love! O sweet and pleasant affection! O pure and sinless intention of the will ... all the more sweet and pleasant for all that is found in it is divine. To reach this state is to become like God. As a drop of water seems to disappear completely in a quantity of wine, even assuming the wine's taste and color; just as red, molten iron becomes so much like fire it seems to lose its primary state ... so it is necessary that all human feelings melt in a mysterious way and flow into the will of God. Otherwise, how will God be all in all if something human survives in man?

— St. Bernard of Clairvaux, *On Loving God*

The Third Power about Holy Sex is that it makes God's own passionate love for each of us physical, tangible, and real. Remember, in Ephesians 5:32 St. Paul tells us that marriage is a sign of Christ's union with his bride, the Church. He calls this "a great mystery." St. Paul doesn't mean "mystery" in the sense that it's a big question mark, but means it in the sense that it reveals a "great and deep truth."

That sex is intended to be a physical sign of God's own passion for each lover is another sense in which sex is sacramental. (The first is the redemptive power I outlined in the last chapter). Catholics are earthy, sensual people. We know that we're bodily creatures, and unlike postmoderns, who value language and spirit over matter, we're not ashamed of it. Because we are bodily creatures, the sacraments always use physical stuff that appeals to our senses and actually makes real what it represents. Or, to use the classical formulation, a sacrament *effects what it signifies*. For instance, the water of baptism *actually washes* the soul clean of original sin. The words of absolution spoken in the sacrament of confession *actually effect* the forgiveness of sin. The bread and wine *actually become* the Body and Blood of our Lord and Savior, Jesus Christ, who becomes our soul's real food and real drink.

Likewise, man and woman — and more particularly, sex — are the actual stuff of the sacrament of marriage. Remember, although service is an essential part of marriage, matrimony itself, as we have already noted, isn't the sacrament of doing dishes together. As Pope John Paul II stated during his 1987 pastoral visit to the United States, "The bond that unites a family is not only a matter of natural kinship or of shared life and experience." Of course, these things are a significant aspect of married life, but marriage itself is the sacrament of sex by which a couple is purified in love and empowered to become co-creators of life with God himself. It is sex that seals and celebrates marriage. If a couple is physically incapable of sex, they cannot complete a valid marriage in the eyes of the Church. The physical love between husband and wife effects what it signifies: the passionate, healing, uniting, and life-giving power of God's love for each of them. Through the sacrament of matrimony, husband and wife are given the responsibility and the grace to be *alteri Christi*, "other Christs," to one another. They are to be the physical sign of how much Christ himself loves each of them. On the days when the couple is so sad, frustrated, careworn, and depleted that they can't imagine that God loves them, the respectful, soulful, selfless lovemaking that rests at the heart of the sacrament of marriage is supposed to empower a husband and wife to look at one another and say, "My spouse loves me so well, I have no doubt of how much God loves me, because no one could love me that much on their own power — in or out of the bedroom."

As Pope John Paul II observed in his reflections on the Theology of the Body, Holy Sex manifests this sacramental sign most powerfully because of its unique capacity to make visible that which is invisible: that is, the passionate desire God has for each person and his longing to be intimately united with each person within a love that is free, faithful, fruitful, and forever. In the act of lovemaking, the couple bears witness in a way that is "a great mystery" — a profound truth — to the intimate, healing, fruitful union God desires with each person.

One of the critical revelations that the Third Power of Holy Sex — the power to image God's love — exposes is that a wife is not a husband's to use as he pleases. Neither is a husband the wife's to use as she pleases. Once married, a husband and wife don't have jurisdiction over their own bodies, but rather belong to one another and are joined in a commitment of mutual generosity (see 1 Cor. 7:4). And God has a prior and primary claim on both the husband and wife. Each and every one of us belongs to God first and foremost (see Rom. 8:14–17). On our own, we count for nothing, but now we are God's people (1 Pet. 2:10). And regardless of the proper hierarchy that exists in Christian marriage, husbands and wives must "defer to one another out of reverence for Christ" (Eph. 5:21), who is the true head of the household and master over both man and woman. As Pope John Paul II wrote in *Familiaris Consortio*:

> *Authentic conjugal love presupposes and requires that a man have a pro-found respect for the equal dignity of his wife: "You are not her master,"* *writes St. Ambrose, "but her husband; she was not given to you to be* *your slave, but your wife. . . . Reciprocate her attentiveness to you and be* *grateful to her for her love." With his wife, a man should live a very* *special form of personal friendship. As for the Christian, he is called* *upon to develop a new attitude of love, manifesting toward his wife a* *charity that is both gentle and strong like that which Christ has for his* *Church.*

Keeping in mind that sex between a husband and wife is a sign of God's own passionate love for both of them, it is essential for husbands and wives to be mindful that they are not just loving each other when they make love. Incredibly, they are the channels through which God himself expresses his desire for passionate union with both husband and wife. This is both an amazing cause for celebration and an incredible responsibility. The husband and the wife must always approach each other with the same passion, joy, abandon, respect, friendship, and care with which God himself loves them. In other words, husband and wife may never use each other as things. Being representatives of God's passion to one another

119

means that a husband and wife may never degrade each other or demand sex as a personal right, duty, or obligation. They must always make certain that their lovemaking occurs in a larger context of mutual generosity, love, and respect.

NAUGHTY, NAUGHTY

The idea that passionate, satisfying lovemaking can also be respectful can come as a surprise to some people. Conventional wisdom asserts that the better sex is, the "naughtier," "dirtier," and "nastier" it has to be. Even counseling professionals fall for this line. In a recent issue of the *Psychotherapy Networker,* a therapist argued that sin is a necessary part of sexy.

C. S. Lewis once referred to England as a nation of apostate Puritans. That is to say, much of Anglo pop-culture is simply a reaction formation to its grimly pious Protestant ancestors. But if England was the cradle of Puritanism, America was its nursery, and we suffer from the same distorted ideas of what constitutes "sin" and being "naughty" as our apostate Puritan cousins across the pond.

As we've discussed previously, Puritans hated sensuality. In their estimation, all the pretty stained glass, incense, vestments, smells, and bells were a papist abomination. As far as they were concerned, you could give them a box to worship in, the Book to read, and one ugly black suit, and they were good to go.

Well, that might be fine for ol' Mom and Dad, but after a while the kids and grandkids got tired of walking around with a big black hat stuck up their rear ends. They started rebelling against the notion that sensuality was sinful. Eventually this led to cultural shifts like the sexual revolution of the 1960s, in which everyone thought they threw over Puritanism for the new girl on the block: hedonism. Really, though, as liberated as secular culture likes to think it is, it can't stop thinking about its Puritan roots, sort of like an estranged oversexed husband who can't overcome his weird obsession with a frigid ex-wife.

In this cultural milieu, it's no wonder people think that sex has to involve "sin" — because they still think sensuality is sinful. "If it feels good it must be bad" — right?

NONSENSE

As any Catholic can tell you, and as we've already established in our discussion of the First Power of Holy Sex, sensuality is an essential ingredient for true spirituality. As far as the Catholic vision of sex is concerned, sex isn't truly spiritual unless it is truly sensual — no sacrament can be, since the whole point of having a sacrament in the first place is so that God can reach us *through our senses*. So if you have bought into the nonsense that sensuality itself is sinful, then yes, sex requires your rather Puritan (and decidedly non-Catholic) sense of sin in order to be sexy.

Of course, there's another sense in which sin is offensive to a healthy sexuality, and that's when one person treats another person as an object, as is the case with pornography or adultery, or when one spouse (physically or emotionally) forces themselves on their mate, or when one spouse insists on sexual acts that are degrading to the dignity of their lover (including contraception). While Catholics don't believe that sensuality is sinful, we do believe that using another person as a means to an end or treating another person in a manner that offends their dignity as a child of God is sinful. It is this authentic sense of sin that is decidedly unsexy.

Husbands and wives must be mad lovers to one another, but they may not be the selfish, objectifying, false lovers held up as examples by our pornographic culture. Rather, spouses must be passionate, godly, mutually respectful, mad lovers as described in the Song of Songs.

> *Groom:* I have come to my garden, my sister, my bride; I gather my myrrh and my spices, I eat my honey and my sweetmeats, I drink my wine and my milk.
>
> *Chorus:* Eat, friends; drink! Drink freely of love!

Bride: I was sleeping, but my heart kept vigil. I heard my lover knocking: "Open to me, my sister, my beloved, my dove, my perfect one." ... My lover put his hand through the opening; my heart trembled within me, and I grew faint when he spoke. I rose to open to my lover, with my hands dripping myrrh: With my fingers dripping choice myrrh upon the fittings of the lock. (Song of Songs 5:1–5)

Is there any question of the passion this couple experiences for one another? And yet, two thousand years of Christian tradition holds that this love poem speaks to both the union between husband and wife and between God and humankind.

Of course, if a couple has an image of God as the punitive, angry, policeman-in-the-sky, then the idea of loving each other as God would love them will be a passion-killing nightmare (but, then, so will heaven). As we discovered previously, this punitive notion of God is simply not Christian — or at least, it isn't Catholic Christian. Such an image has more to do with the god of the Jansenists, who never learned to smile. When a couple has a healthy, Catholic vision of God as a joyful, gentle, passionate, respectful lover, the couple can discover a freedom that allows them to experience a sensual, free, fruitful, abundant, playful, joyful sexual relationship without fear of using each other, degrading each other, or diminishing each other.

BEVERLY AND SAM'S STORY

Beverly and Sam have been married ten years. They have three children. They met in college, and shortly after they began dating they attended an event hosted by the campus featuring a popular speaker on the theology of the body.

"I thought I knew everything worth knowing about sex," says Sam, "but that talk really opened my eyes to what God was trying to tell a couple through their bodies. I'd never heard anything like it."

Beverly adds, "Of course, I'd always known sex was about love. But I thought it was mainly about two people who loved each other making each other feel good. It never occurred to me that it meant more than that."

The Janus Report on sexuality observed that religious people report better sexual relationships than nonreligious partners because of their ability to appreciate the spiritual dimensions of sexuality. Sam and Beverly found this to be the case when they got married a year later and began to experience the divine power of Holy Sex.

"We'd both been sexually active in our early college years," says Sam, "but we decided that we wanted to wait for marriage to make love to each other. Maybe it sounds corny, but I don't really care if it does. Once we learned how precious sex really was, we wanted to wait to give ourselves to each other in the right way at the right time. It was hard."

Beverly seconds that. "Sometimes it was really difficult, but waiting got us off to a great start. I think when any couple makes love for the first time, you can be a little tentative, but from the beginning we were just more open with each other than we had ever been with anyone else because we knew God was loving us through each other."

"That might freak some people out," Sam says, "but it opened us up to each other in a big way."

"It freed me up to push myself to try new ways to be more passionate and show Sam how much I love him," says Sara, "because I wasn't just loving him on my own power. And I think it gave us a way of challenging each other if we ever felt uneasy about something or were worried we were taking advantage of each other. We'd just ask if the way we were acting toward each other was the way God would want to show us he loved us."

Sam picks it up from here, "Sometimes one of us would want to make love when the other didn't or try a position that the other wasn't sure about, but since it wasn't anything immoral and we work hard to be loving to each other throughout the day, we were able to say, 'Yeah, this risk you're asking me to take is safe. It's worth it.' And sometimes, it'd be clear that something one of us wanted to do just wasn't all right because it didn't really help us connect with God's love."

Other couples genuinely struggle when it comes to communicating their needs, desires, and feelings about sex and negotiating whether certain acts are acceptable or which spouse's ideas regarding frequency are "correct." But as Beverly and Sam's story shows, when a couple is mindful that they are sharing God's love for each other and not just their own, it gives them a way to challenge unreasonable barriers to intimacy and assert necessary boundaries that protect the dignity of each person. That makes the vulnerability required in healthy lovemaking safe, and the sexual relationship itself joyful.

TOPPLING THE BARRIERS TO INTIMACY

All this leads to the question, "What's the secret to celebrating the kind of love that, rooted in God's love for the couple, has the power to topple unnecessary barriers to intimacy while safeguarding the dignity of the husband and wife?" In other words, how do we love with God's love, which is both all-consumingly passionate and deeply respectful? The key is always remembering that your beloved is a person toward whom the only logical response is authentic, godly love. Catholic philosophers call this statement "the personalistic norm." It is so easy to forget that people are really persons. It's so easy to think of people as means to ends, as things that I can use to make my life easier or more pleasant. Have you ever been treated like an object? Perhaps a friend of yours calls you only when he wants to borrow your tools, or when she had another fight with her husband. Maybe your cousin gets in touch only when she needs money, or maybe your spouse ignores you until he (or she) wants to make love or go on a date, or buy a new trinket for the house. It feels awful, doesn't it? In such times, you probably feel degraded, resentful, humiliated, and angry. And really, you *should* feel that way, because you're being used. At any rate, even if you give in to the request, the experience doesn't endear you to the other person. Rather than enjoying the opportunity to share your gifts and treasure to make someone else's life better, you might feel used and might become more stingy with others — whether or not they deserve it — as a way of protecting yourself. In other words, the experience of being used in little and big ways diminishes you.

124

In *Love and Responsibility*, Karol Wojtyla argued that the opposite of love is not hate. Rather, the opposite of loving someone is using someone. To love someone is to work for that person's good. To love someone is to place that person's interests, joys, and needs first. That doesn't mean that you can't get what you want out of your life and relationships; it just means that you can never try to get what you want in a way that "thing-ifies" the person you are asking to meet that need or desire. Manifesting God's love to your beloved means being careful of the constant temptation to treat someone as an object, or a means to an end, instead of a person toward whom the only proper response is true love.

Becoming an Infallible Lover means striving to become the kind of person who works, every day, to help your mate become the person God created him or her to be. Whether you feel like it or not. Holy Sex requires you to convey to your mate every single day that you're the person who will do anything — especially things that challenge your comfort zone — to help your mate live the fullest, most joyful, most meaningful, intimate, and virtuous life possible.

As we saw earlier, the premier marriage researcher in the country, Dr. John Gottman, evaluated couples to find out what makes good marriages good and other marriages not so good. He discovered that the couples whose relationships are the best, most intimate, most affectionate, and most fulfilling were those couples who maintained a 20:1 ratio of positive to negative interactions with each other throughout their relationship and a 5:1 ratio of positivity to negativity in arguments. These so-called "marriage masters" were twenty times more complimentary, supportive, encouraging, affectionate, and self-sacrificing than they were complaining, criticizing, argumentative, or nagging.

None of this is to say that these "masters of marriage" are always syrupy-sweet with each other. Sometimes they argue. Sometimes they have complaints. They aren't always perfectly happy with each other. But they are always supportive, and they always look for ways to make each other's lives easier or more pleasant. And in arguments, they try to make sure that they work on the problem together and never treat each other as if the other is the problem. These couples know that, as important as it is to solve problems, it's more important to take care of your teammate.

This is the personalistic norm at work. This is what it takes to celebrate Holy Sex: that toe-curling, mind-blowing, eye-popping, deeply spiritual, and profoundly sanctifying sexuality that takes the love God holds in his heart for you and your mate and manifests it physically.

HI HO, HI HO — WORKING AT YOUR RELATIONSHIP

There is yet another dimension to loving each other with God's love that has implications for the married couple's sexual relationship and the rest of the marriage. This is the willingness to work on the relationship for the sake of achieving the greatest unity and intimacy humanly possible.

Some people believe that relationships, if they are good, should "just happen." This often goes double for people's ideas about sexual relationships, since the world speaks so much about the importance of "chemistry" with regard to sex. The truth is that the kind of passionate, fulfilling, soulful, godly, lifelong sexual relationship to which Infallible Lovers aspire takes real work.

This is a passion killer for people who place too much faith in their hormones as the source of sexual intimacy, but Infallible Lovers take as their model the Mad, Divine Lover. They recognize that if God, who really doesn't need us after all, is willing to go through such lengths as emptying himself, being born a man, suffering the indignities of childhood and the meanness of daily life, risking rejection by those he loves, and suffering the most humiliating and painful death on a cross all for the sake of winning our hearts, what could we not be willing to do for the sake of our beloved?

Infallible Lovers recall the parable of the unmerciful servant (Matt. 18:21–25), who, having been forgiven the huge debt he owed his king, proceeded to beat up one of his own friends for what amounted to lunch money. In the same way, Infallible Lovers recognize that if God is willing to work so hard on his relationship with us, we must also be willing to work to achieve the closest intimacy possible with our mate both in and out of the bedroom.

Many other faiths are primarily about creeds and doctrine. While Christianity also has creeds and doctrines that require assent if one wishes to be considered a member of the communion, Christianity is not so much a set of creeds as a relationship with the Person of Jesus Christ and the communion of saints. Through Christ, God calls us, not primarily to profess a doctrine, but to be in an intimate union with him. This is even more true about Catholicism, which believes that God's desire for union with his people is so intense that he would go through the trouble of instituting the sacrament of the Eucharist. Catholics believe that God doesn't just love us for our minds. He wants union with our bodies too. He wants us to be part of his own flesh and blood. "Unless you eat of the flesh of the Son of Man and drink of his blood, you shall have no life in you" (John 6:53–63).

This is the kind of intimacy to which the Infallible Lover is called, and this takes a willingness to work hard for the sake of celebrating authentic love. Let lesser lovers lazily roll off a log and fall into bed with one another. Infallible Lovers, who long to celebrate the fullness of Holy Sex, are willing to challenge themselves daily to leave behind their comfort zones to love their mate — not just the way they want to love their mate, but in the manner *their mate says* they need to be loved. All day long, in and out of the bedroom, Infallible Lovers, confirmed in the desire to love each other with God's own passion, are willing to do whatever it takes (short of offending their own dignity or God's moral laws) and leave behind whatever personal comforts and preferences may stand in the way of loving their beloved in a manner that makes sense to the beloved.

When a husband and wife exemplify such profound respect for and commitment to one another, they activate the Third Power of Holy Sex: the ability to take the invisible reality of God's passionate love for each lover and make it visible. Practicing Holy Sex empowers a couple to celebrate the kind of epic love story told in the Song of Songs. Holy Sex gives every married couple what it takes to turn their marriage into a love poem that bonds man and woman, weds heaven and earth, and inspires generations of lovers with the authentic power of godly passion.

Intrigued? Good. We'll discuss more ways to turn up this kind of love in your home in chapter 13. But now it's time to turn our attention to the next truth about Holy Sex.

$\mathcal{8}$ SEX UNITES

It is not good for man to be alone.
—Genesis 2:10

Every single one of us feels incomplete on our own. As you see from the epigraph at the beginning of this chapter, Scripture asserts the incompleteness of the solitary person. Enter the Fourth Power of Holy Sex to the rescue: sex unites!

Holy Sex unites! Holy Sex has the power to take two hearts and melt them into one, body and soul (Matt. 19:5). When couples practice Holy Sex, lovemaking becomes both an instrument and a sign of their one-ness.

In his *Theology of the Body*, Pope John Paul II reminded us that in order to discern God's intentions for the relationship between man and woman, Jesus tells us that we must go back to the beginning — that is, to God's Word in Genesis. In the beginning, we are told that woman was created out of man. Contrary to what secular feminists might tell you, this does not mean that woman is somehow an afterthought or less than man. For the Catholic Christian, it means that, unlike religions where women represent the lesser sex, woman was made of the same biological, psychological, emotional, relational, and spiritual stuff as man. In Eve, Adam saw a perfect helpmate and partner. Pope John Paul II argued that before the Fall, man, woman, and God experienced "original unity," a perfect harmony and intimate connection rooted in God's love, mutual service, intimate understanding, and respect.

The fact that woman was made from man also means that man is missing part of himself, and that only through union with woman will he ever be whole. "This is why man leaves his father and mother and cleaves to his wife and they shall become one flesh" (Gen. 2:24). The union between husband and wife is stronger even than the union between mother and son (much to the anguish of mothers everywhere) because it is through the sexual union between husband and wife that the two, in a sense, discover the missing aspects of themselves.

After the regrettable apple incident (a.k.a. "The Fall"), the original unity enjoyed between man, woman, and God was ruptured. Man and woman became self-focused rather than other-focused. Over time, man and woman came to think of each other almost as separate species, beings from two different planets who can barely understand each other, much less relate to each other. The regrettable apple incident was to the communion of man and woman what the Tower of Babel was to the communion of nations.

But this way of being is a lie. This is not the way it was intended to be "in the beginning," and it's not the way God intends it to be now. That is why God raised marriage to the dignity of a sacrament and reasserted the power that sex had at the beginning of time to be an instrument of sacred union between man and woman and God. Some readers may be thinking, "This is a lovely religious myth and all, but this just isn't reality."

Some readers would be wrong.

If the Christian claim is true that sex was intended by God as an instrument of unity from the beginning of creation, then there should be evidence of this in our created, physical being. And there is. Science shows that lovemaking actually physically bonds two people together, not merely in a romantic, spiritual, or even psychological sense, but *physically* as well. When a man and woman make love, chemicals such as oxytocin (in both men and women) and vasopressin (in men) are released into the body. These chemicals, among others, actually create a physical bond between the lovers. They have the effect of making the couple miss each other and long for one another. They enable the couple to tolerate petty offenses more easily. They increase feelings of trust between the lovers. They reduce fear and increase a desire for vulnerability.

Holy Sex truly marries two people to one another. It makes them physiologically crave one another. The lover in the Song of Solomon cries out,

"Set me as a seal on your heart!" (Song of Songs 8:6). Holy Sex literally and physically stamps the lovers with each other's impression, causing them to ache to be one. The lovers in the Song of Songs crave one another when they are apart.

> *By night on my bed I sought him whom my soul loves: I sought him, but I found him not. I said, I will rise now, and go about the city; In the streets and in the broad ways I will seek him whom my soul loves: I sought him, but I found him not. The watchmen that go about the city found me; To whom I said, Have you seen him whom my soul loves? It was but a little that I passed from them, When I found him whom my soul loves: I held him, and would not let him go.*

The lovers of the Song of Songs crave each other so deeply that it inspires utterly insane behavior. In a culture that frowns upon women traveling unchaperoned, a lone woman goes forth, at night, risking her safety and her reputation (after all, in this culture what sort of women wander around unattended at night?) to make a fool of herself by begging the local constabulary — who have plenty of other more important things to do — to help her find the man who has barely been gone from her side. She aches for him, and we ache for our beloved, not just because we psychologically enjoy our beloved's company, but because our bodies were made to *need* each other.

THE CHEMISTRY OF SEX

Advances in brain scanning technology have given rise to a new discipline called "interpersonal neurobiology." This is the study of how relationships actually change the brains of the people involved in them. In *A General Theory of Love,* the physicians and co-authors Thomas Lewis, Fari Amini, and Richard Lannon assert: "When somebody loses a partner, and says that part of him is gone, he is more right than he thinks. A portion of his neural activity depends on the presence of that other living brain."

Scientists now know that, far from being mere recreation, sex is a process that physiologically bonds two people to one another by altering both brain chemistry and brain function in the lovers. Some of these changes occur the first time a couple makes love. The longer a couple is together, the more their brains change and come into synch with each other. Brain researchers know that romantic love stimulates at least three specific major parts of the brain: the caudate nucleus, the anterior cingulate gyrus, and the insular cortex.

WHAT IT ALL MEANS FOR YOU

Jenny and Bill are newlyweds. They can barely stand to be apart. The other day, Bill got in trouble with his boss for calling Jenny for the tenth time that day just to hear her voice. He knows he's being silly. He just misses her and can't wait to get home to her again.

The caudate nucleus is the brain's reward center. It's the part of the brain that says, "I've found something wonderful! Give me more of that!" Research shows that the caudate nucleus continues to be stimulated over the duration of an intimate relationship, but it fires the strongest in the early stages of romantic, sexual love, compelling the lovers to stick together until deeper bonding can occur.

It's been a rough day. Madelyn was raked over the coals by a client at work, and the kids seem like their teacher injected them with a hypodermic needle full of sugar water and amphetamines. What were they doing in school today anyway? She glances at the small picture of Jim she keeps on the dashboard and feels a flood of warm feelings. God, she can't wait for him to hold her again.

The anterior cingulate gyrus is responsible for things like anticipating rewards, enhancing empathy, and producing warm, positive emotions. This part of the brain does not fire as intensely in the early stages of love, but it fires more and more strongly the longer two lovers are together. Scientists believe this is the part of the brain that makes you feel that deep warmth toward your spouse, compels you to take care of your mate, and anticipates the feeling of wholeness you get every time he or she walks into the room.

It's 2:30 a.m., but Lily is awake. Her husband, James, is on a business trip, and she can never sleep well when he's not there. She chides herself for being silly. You'd think after fifteen years of marriage you would be glad to get rid of each other once in a while. Suddenly her heart leaps into her throat as the phone rings. Who could it be? What could be wrong? It's James.

He couldn't sleep either.

Finally, the insular cortex appears to be the seat of the deepest bonding between husband and wife. Like the anterior cingulate gyrus, it becomes more active the longer one person is in relationship with another. Its job is to evaluate how the different organs and systems in your body feel. This part of the brain causes you to ache when your partner is away for long periods, to feel butterflies when you're sharing a moment of playful affection, or to feel terribly sick when faced with the possibility of losing your mate to disease, death, or divorce.

These are only a few of the ways lovers actually stamp their impressions onto each other's physical being and ultimately become one with each other emotionally, spiritually, and physically. When the Bible tells us that "the two shall become one" (Matt. 19:5) or warns against casual sex by saying that we become joined to our sexual partner (1 Cor. 6:16), it isn't just speaking metaphorically. You really do become one flesh with a person with whom you have sex. And the longer you're in a physically intimate relationship, the deeper the bond becomes.

As a side note, promiscuous sex actually impedes a lover's ability to subsequently bond with a partner. Break-ups actually trigger the same pain centers of the brain that light up when you suffer physical trauma. Our bodies were simply not intended to have multiple sexual partners. When couples have sex and break up, it's the neurobiological equivalent of taking a hammer and beating the dickens out of the plug at the end of your radio power cord and then trying to insert it into a wall socket.

Depending on how hard and how often you hit that plug, you may not be able to make a real connection at all. And even if you can plug it in, the connection may be fragile. While a plug that hasn't been abused can stand a little jostling, the hammered-on plug doesn't hold up as well, and may snap off in the wall too easily, breaking the connection. Neurobiologically speaking, when other factors are equal, two people who are virgins at marriage have the greatest potential of forging the strongest bond — a bond that can withstand the jostling of the relationship that comes with conflict and the trials of life. The more promiscuous members of a couple were before marriage, the weaker — biologically speaking — the physical bond will be. This may lead to the more sexually experienced couple being less able to tolerate the normal stresses and strains of married life.

There is a wide body of research supporting this notion. For instance, attachment scientists (researchers who study how human pair bonds are made between children and parents as well as adult lovers) know that when humans — whether children or adults — repeatedly make and break pair bonds (between children and caregivers or, in adulthood, between sexual partners), the condition known as "defensive attachment" will develop. Defensive attachment is the brain's way of defending itself from rejection. While the person who exhibits healthy attachment experiences joy and longing in the presence of a lover, the person with defensive attachment experiences a physiological sense of numbness in the presence of an intimate partner. The person who suffers from defensive attachment projects an "I don't need anybody" or "I don't care if you care" attitude in a relationship that makes intimacy more and more difficult. Each previous broken pair-bond (e.g., failed caregiving relationship in childhood or failed sexual relationship in adulthood) exacerbates this condition. In the extreme, defensive attachment problems become reactive attachment problems, which can prevent a person from ever risking the vulnerability necessary for a healthy relationship. The good news is that defensive attachment can be healed, but it takes a great deal of work and a willingness to consciously challenge the very strong, very real, gut-level sense that vulnerability, trust, and intimacy are dangerous.

Sex Unites

The case against multiple sexual partners can also be made from research on factors that predict divorce. A 2003 study appearing in the *Journal of Marriage and the Family* studied a representative sample of women from the National Survey of Family Growth and found that women who had multiple sexual partners before marriage experienced a significantly higher rate of divorce than women who were virgins at marriage. Likewise, the study showed that the more partners a person had before marriage, the greater the risk of divorce. While no doubt many psychological factors play into this reality, one should not underestimate the fact that the more sexual partners a person has, the weaker the physical bond that is created between subsequent lovers, and the harder it becomes to create a successful, intimate bond with one's lover in the first place.

LOVE UNWRAPPED

This discussion leads to another important point you've probably never considered. In light of the power of sex to unite two people physiologically, it's highly likely that barrier methods of contraception (such as condoms) actually inhibit the depth of long-term bonding by muting the chemical reactions and brain changes that result when the man ejaculates inside the woman. The presence of semen in the vagina causes a powerful chemical chain reaction in the woman, and the absence of this chemical reaction cannot help but impede the physiological process of attachment of one lover to another. Even laying aside the decreased physical sensations that accompany intercourse with a condom, the impaired chemical bond could also account for the fact that many couples using barrier methods report that lovemaking is simply not as satisfying as intercourse without the physical barrier. Not only are those who have a love affair with latex depriving their senses, but they're starving their bodies of the union that each physically craves with the other.

Think it doesn't really matter? Think of it this way. Consider the number of times a married couple will make love over the years. If the average happy couple has sex four times a month and is married around fifty years,

135

that couple will have sexual intercourse around twenty-four hundred or more times over the course of their lifetime together. Compare the cumulative effect of hundreds of these less satisfying condom-contained sexual encounters with the cumulative effect of the same number of considerably more rewarding, latex-free experiences, and you begin to see how couples cheat themselves when they use condoms. Just to drive my point home, if you did twenty-four hundred sets of sit-ups, wouldn't you expect it to have an effect on your body? What about running up twenty-four hundred flights of stairs? I'll bet you'd feel that.

But what if rather than doing sit-ups twenty-four hundred times, someone simply pulled you into a sitting position twenty-four hundred times? Or what if instead of running up the stairs, you simple rode up and down in an elevator twenty-four hundred times? Would your body be as fit as the person who experienced the fullness of the exercise?

If these physical activities are expected to have a physical effect on your body, and if avoiding these activities has an effect on your body, why wouldn't lovemaking, which is nothing if not a physical act, also have a cumulative effect on your body? And wouldn't the couple who allowed themselves to experience the full chemical and physical union of intercourse experience a greater benefit to their bond than those who deprived themselves in some way?

When the Church teaches that barrier methods of contraception (as well as other forms of artificial birth control) offend the uniting power of sex, the Church may be speaking more literally — and, considering our emerging understanding of interpersonal neurobiological processes, more profoundly — than most people think.

A UNION OF SPIRITS

Sex clearly has a deep and literal power both to draw people into a closer relationship with each other and to make them want to be a stronger and more profound influence in each other's lives. This is where the psychological and spiritual aspects of physiological bonding occur. St. Paul's caution against intimate relationships with unbelievers (see 2 Cor. 6:14) takes on new significance when one truly understands that one person becomes neurochemically and physiologically dependent upon another person over time. Psychologists know that the stronger the physical and emotional attachment between two people, the more alike they also become in values, beliefs, and morals. This dimension of normal, human attachment behavior is called identification. It refers to the strong drive to look more and be more like the people with whom I experience a sense of belonging.

The unitive power of love is a double-edged sword in this regard. If you are a believing spouse and strong in your faith, the unitive power of your sexual relationship may ultimately result in the sanctification of your unbelieving mate (see 1 Cor. 7:14), as the increasing attachment between you both challenges your mate to seek out your values. By contrast, if you are not as strong in your faith, that faith can easily be undermined by the attachment that forms between you and your lover, causing you to make more and more exceptions and allowances for the sake of the nonbeliever, leading you both to spiritual ruin. I've seen this ruin many times, including in the case of Gina, a woman I counseled.

GINA AND JOHN'S STORY

Gina and John have been married twenty years. They have two children — one in college and the other a high school sophomore. John was raised in a nonreligious home. Gina's family attended church and, as an adult, so did Gina. She even served as a reader at Mass. She considered herself a good Christian — not a fanatic, mind you — but she felt that her faith was significant. Although the intellectual and deeper spiritual aspects of her faith were largely underdeveloped, her involvement in church remained personally important to her.

John has no real interest in religion. He isn't hostile to it. He just doesn't care. His attitude is that if Gina wants to go to Mass, that's fine with him as long as she leaves him out of it. He considers himself a good man. He prays in his own way and doesn't feel the need for some ritual to get close to God. God is important to John. It's just that John doesn't have any need to be "one of those crazy people who goes to church all the time." He has no desire to have anyone tell him what to do. He's a grown-up, after all. For the most part, there is little conflict around matters of faith in the couple's day-to-day relationship.

Recently, John has been complaining to Gina that their sex life is stagnant. He began suggesting that they watch pornography together as a way of "spicing things up" and "getting some new ideas." Gina was initially resistant. She knew that the Church frowns on pornography, but it wouldn't be like watching some disgusting movie in a filthy theater by herself somewhere. There were tasteful sexual videos, weren't there? She didn't exactly feel right about it, but she couldn't place her finger on why, except that maybe there was some lingering prudery hanging around from something she heard the nuns say at some point or another. She decided she was being silly. She loves John and wants to make him happy. So, laying down some guidelines about the kinds of things she wasn't willing to see, she told John that she would be willing to watch the videos with him.

The results were decidedly mixed. On the one hand, the videos did arouse the couple, and they did become more experimental in their sexual relationship. Things certainly did seem more exciting in some ways. Still, Gina would often find herself wondering what John was thinking about when he closed his eyes when they were making love. Was he imagining the women on the videos? Could she keep up with them? Physically, things seemed better, but emotionally, she just didn't feel as close to John as she'd hoped she would.

One day John came home from work and shared that some friends of his from work regularly went to a local "gentlemen's club" with their wives. They said it was harmless fun and that being in that environment really turned up the volume on their own sex lives at home. Gina was appalled at first, but she didn't have access to any well-formed religious or intellectual reasons to object. She just knew what she felt. Of course, she loved John and wanted to do anything that could make him happy. But she just felt it was wrong.

John pushed back. In the face of her inability to articulate any solid reasons why she shouldn't go to the club, he accused her of being uptight and acting "holier than thou." Didn't she want to have fun? Why was she so ashamed of the body? Didn't she want the best sexual relationship they could have? Why was she letting her religion get in the way of their marriage? What was more important — the approval of a bunch of allegedly celibate old pervs who were too interested in altar boys to know anything about real love, or her love for her husband?

Gina knew John had her there. She still felt funny about the whole thing, but John seemed so adamant. Although she enjoyed sex, she knew that John had always placed an especially heavy emphasis on their sexual relationship, and in the early years they'd had a lot of arguments about frequency and such. She didn't want to lose him, and she did want to show him she loved him. What would it hurt, really? Maybe she should just grow up and stop holding on to that religious guilt. God didn't really care what she and John did in their bedroom, as long as they really loved each other — right?

Gina and John got together with his friends the following Saturday night and went to the local gentlemen's club. Gina was surprised. The place was nicer than she'd imagined. It was tastefully furnished. And the show was really professional. In spite of herself, Gina found herself imagining doing for John some of the things she was watching the women doing. She imagined how happy she would make him, and that made her happy and aroused. Sure, she felt a little guilty about being there, and she wasn't sure how she really felt about John staring at other women, but wasn't that just because she was holding on to childish ideas about sex? It wasn't like he was going alone to strip clubs. He wanted her there with him. This was for their marriage. Surely she was mature enough to handle this. That night, to take the edge off her nerves, she had a little more to drink than usual, and she felt the tension melt away. She started enjoying herself. Toward the end of the evening, she started making out with John right there at the table. She whispered in his ear that he should take her home. They only made it halfway home before they stopped in the parking lot of a closed grocery store and had sex in the car. They felt like naughty teenagers.

Gina and John started getting together with their strip-club friends more often, and their physical relationship was more intense than ever. But in spite of everything, she couldn't shake the feeling that she was losing him — that somehow, he wasn't really with her even when he was with her. She didn't know why. Maybe she was crazy. Things were great, right?

Eventually Gina learned to quiet that inner voice that kept nagging her that John was someplace else. Even though she was still a little conflicted, everything seemed great, so what was she worried about? Wasn't she a freer person than ever? God still loved her. She was sure of it. Why shouldn't he? She was a good person. And John seemed happy.

That's why it was such a surprise to her when John announced that he'd fallen in love with Kate — one of the women they had been going clubbing with. They had been planning for months.

Gina had always been somewhat fascinated and somewhat uncomfortable with Kate, a woman who was just so "out there" in the provocative way she dressed and how sexually assertive she was. Kate seemed like a nice woman with a good heart, but she could be crazy too. One time, she actually got up and danced with one of the strippers at the club. Gina and the other wives who went to the strip clubs together were never sure whether to think of Kate as a role model — the other husbands seemed to want their wives to be more like Kate — or to be wary of her. Now Gina knew. John left Gina that day and moved in with the other woman. Gina was devastated. She felt like an idiot. Why couldn't she see it coming? For his part, John said he was sorry to hurt Gina (though he didn't seem terribly remorseful) but "it just happened."

About a year after the divorce, Gina moved in with another man she met through an online dating service. She says she's happy, but doesn't ever want to marry again. She says she doesn't want to let anybody hurt her like that again.

HEALTHY AND DEFENSIVE ATTACHMENT

Why couldn't Gina see it coming? Two answers. First, she was not formed well enough in her own faith to be able to offer objective reasons (other than "it's bad" or "it feels wrong") why she didn't want to go down the road John wanted to take her. Second, she ached when she imagined losing John. She was physically bonded to John and couldn't stand the thought of not having him in her life. That bond easily trumped the meaningful, but rather shallow, emotional connection she had to her faith. For the sake of maintaining the physical bond created by sex, Gina became more like John and ended up as shallow as John despite herself. (Note: Gina and John's situation is a good example of defensive attachment.)

I want to emphasize that the problem in Gina and John's relationship was not their sensuality. If a couple wishes to experiment with different sexual positions, wear lingerie, tell each other provocative things, make love in the back of the car, or be passionately affectionate, by all means they should do so. Holy Sex is sensual sex, after all. The problem with John and Gina was that they pursued sensuality without respect for each other's dignity as children of God, without respect for the integrity of the marriage, and without respect for the fact that sensuality cannot be pursued as an end in itself. It can only be pursued as a means of revealing God's love for each lover. In this way, a couple who long to be Infallible Lovers can have a passionate and even erotic sexual life that is rooted in mutual respect for each other, the integrity of the marriage, and God's plan for their lives.

One way or the other, the two will become one. Whether that is for good or ill depends largely on the character strength of the individual spouses and the appropriate spiritual support they are able to find to keep them on the path that leads to their Divine Lover.

In situations where both the husband and the wife are faithful, however, it's easy to imagine how their growing bond and deeper attachment to one another can create a powerfully synergistic spiritual reality. Such a couple can help each other grow as neither could on his or her own. The relationship between Jack and Marylin, married twenty-four years with four children, is an excellent example of this dynamic.

JACK AND MARYLIN'S STORY

Jack and Marylin were both faithful Catholics when they got married in college. They met at the Newman Center, regularly attended Mass together, and were active in various social justice causes. Sexually, their interests were generally compatible. As the years went by, they would challenge each other to grow spiritually and relationally in ways that were difficult but rewarding for both.

Jack, for his part, had a long-term struggle with his temper. "I would never become violent with Marylin, but I'd slam doors and curse. Things like that. I never meant to be intimidating, but I was. There were lots of times Marylin and the kids felt like they had to tiptoe around me."

Over the years, Jack and Marylin worked hard to improve their relationship. They prayed together more often, went on marriage retreats to learn better communication, and tried to look for ways to care for one another in their day-to-day relationship. Although Jack had never thought of these things as his cup of tea, he loved Marylin, and as they grew closer together, over time, he wanted to find ways to be a better man for her. In time, Jack felt challenged more and more to let go of his anger. As Jack puts it, "I just realized how stupid it was. I wasn't being the person I felt like God wanted me to be. But I have to say I'd already known that for a long time, and it didn't really motivate me to change. What finally did it was that I felt like Marylin deserved better. Her love made me want to give up my tantrums. I wanted to love her better."

Marylin, on the other hand, struggled with affection. "I wasn't raised in a real affectionate home, y'know? I knew my mom and dad loved me, but they didn't really show it very much. Not to me or anybody."

Jack, who was as passionate about showing affection as he was about showing his anger, often felt frozen out emotionally by Marylin in the early years of their relationship. After they had children, Jack continued to be concerned that Marylin was holding back from them too. As Marylin explains, "We used to have terrible arguments about how John felt I wasn't giving either him or our kids the love they deserved. I just felt like he wanted me to be someone I wasn't. But the longer we were together, the more I saw how people — especially the kids — just glowed when Jack was around. I wanted to be able to do that for people. I wanted to be able to give that to him, not just in the bedroom but in all parts of our lives. It's been hard work, but I've really come a long way. I'm a lot more affectionate than I ever thought I'd be comfortable with. The more Jack got control of his temper, the safer I felt around him, and the more I was able to see how much he really works hard to serve me and the family. I've been a lot more open to his suggestions to try different positions and be more playful in lovemaking. He's helped me become a lot more assertive about what pleases me, *too, and we're closer than ever — emotionally and sexually. I'm really grateful for Jack's patience and love. It made me want to give him my best."*

Jack and Marylin are a good example of how the unitive power of love can challenge two faithful people to want to be more for each other and for God. God hard-wires human beings to attach to one another and be able to influence one another, so that together they can become much more than they could ever be on their own. That's the unitive power of marriage at work.

When we compare the previous case of Gina and John with the case of Jack and Marylin, we see a clear illustration of what Pope Benedict XVI wrote in his encyclical *Deus Caritas Est* (God is love).

> Eros, *reduced to pure "sex," has become a commodity, a mere "thing" to be bought and sold, or rather, man himself becomes a commodity. This is hardly man's great "yes" to the body. On the contrary, he now considers his body and his sexuality as the purely material part of himself, to be used and exploited at will. Nor does he see it as an arena for the exercise of his freedom, but as a mere object that he attempts, as he pleases, to make both enjoyable and harmless. Here we are actually dealing with a debasement of the human body: no longer is it integrated into our overall existential freedom; no longer is it a vital expression of our whole being, but it is more or less relegated to the purely biological sphere. The apparent exaltation of the body can quickly turn into a hatred of bodiliness. Christian faith, on the other hand, has always considered man a unity in duality, a reality in which spirit and matter compenetrate, and in which each is brought to a new nobility. True eros tends to rise "in ecstasy" toward the Divine, to lead us beyond ourselves; yet for this very reason it calls for a path of ascent, renunciation, purification, and healing.*

The union of Gina and John led, despite their intentions, to their mutual debasement and the disintegration of their marriage, while the union of Jack and Marylin made a proper use of erotic love. By rooting their passion in the context of their larger relationship and founding it on principles of mutual respect, they were able to allow eros to help them "rise in ecstasy toward the Divine."

When a couple celebrates the Fourth Truth, the uniting power of sex, they create a bond that imprints the very essence of each lover upon the other's body and soul. The Fourth Power of Holy Sex, the power to unite the two into one, forges a physiological, emotional, and spiritual bond between lovers that cannot be broken by God or man. "What God has joined, let no one tear apart" (Matt. 19:6).

9 SEX CREATES

Man cannot find himself except by making a sincere gift of himself.
— *Gaudium et Spes*

When a man and woman consciously and of their own free will choose to marry and have sexual relations, they choose at the same time the possibility of procreation. . . . And it is only when they do so that they put their sexual relationship within the framework of marriage on a truly personal level. — Karol Wojtyla, *Love and Responsibility*

The Fifth Power of Holy Sex is the most amazing and mysterious of all the Five Powers. It is the power to create. Holy Sex challenges lovers to see that the incredible power of their love for each other cannot be kept between the two of them. Holy Sex seeks to celebrate a love that is so powerful that in nine months it has to be given its own name. Holy Sex taps into the creative spark of Divine Love that longs to create more creatures to love and allows men and women to glimpse the joy God himself experiences when his love bursts into life.

Since the sexual revolution and the advent of the first effective, mass market contraceptive pill, sex has largely come to be seen as a primarily recreational exercise. But for over two hundred thousand years of human history prior to the sexual revolution, sex was understood to be the pleasurable means by which children are brought into the world and the survival of the species was assured. In short, we, the product of all these many millennia of evolutionary improvement, represent the first generations of humankind so stupid as to actually be shocked — and even, in some cases, appalled — when sex causes babies. We've completely forgotten that this is actually the way it is supposed to be. Honest. Really. No, I'm not kidding.

While our *I'm-way-too-sexy-for-this-body* postmodern culture sniffs that humankind has evolved beyond the need to worry about such ridiculous biological imperatives as the propagation of the human race, Mother Nature proves, once again, that it is she who laughs both last and best.

For years, doomsayers, inspired by the work of Stanford professor Paul Erlich, fretted about the so-called "population bomb," crusading against reason to assert that the only way humanity could save itself was to cease perpetuating itself. In the scarcely two generations that have followed the social re-jiggering required to prevent the alleged Great Baby Catastrophe, contraception has become *de rigueur,* and childbearing is the counter-cultural phenom on the world stage. The result is that many countries — in Western Europe particularly — are flirting with economic and social collapse as the comparatively few children born since the 1970s struggle to support an aging population and the social institutions the previous generation created to accommodate its numbers. Demographers suggest that America may not be far behind.

The West isn't the only beneficiary of the "Gospel of Planned Barren-hood." In the East, China's draconian one-child policy has resulted in decades of genocide against female babies. (They could have used a hand from those who consider themselves secular feminist freedom fighters.) As a result, present and future generations of young Chinese men are unable to find women to marry.

Pope Paul VI prophetically predicted these population problems back in 1967, years before they began:

> *Who will blame a government which in its attempt to resolve the problems affecting an entire country resorts to the same measures as are regarded as lawful by married people in the solution of a particular family difficulty? Who will prevent public authorities from favoring those contraceptive methods which they consider more effective? Should they regard this as necessary, they may even impose their use on everyone.* (Humanae Vitae)

And the results of all this social engineering have been disastrous. Whether we care to admit it or not, we can't escape the reality that we are biological creatures who will always need to honor our biological roots — or pay the price. As Catholic social critic Mark Shea is fond of saying, "All of human history can be summed up in two sentences: First, 'What could it hurt?' Followed sometime after by, 'How was I supposed to know?'"

The contemporary Cult of Barrenness is bearing bad fruit a little closer to home as well. In her book *The Good Marriage*, marriage researcher Judith Wallerstein describes an emerging phenomenon she calls "the Romantic Anti-Marriage." This relationship, rather than being a vital, loving, healthy union, is an insular, ultimately suffocating relationship in which the couple becomes narcissistically focused on each other, squeezing out the rest of the world, including children. According to Wallerstein's research, such a couple lacks the capacity for a good marriage because they lack the maturity to step outside of themselves, not simply for the sake of themselves or children, but for each other's sake as well.

Openness to life is an essential part of a mature sexuality. I don't mean "mature" in the euphemistic sense of "old, stodgy, and requiring the assistance of a walker and an iron lung." I mean in the way a flower in full bloom is mature, or a wine at the peak of its vintage is mature.

The joyfully mature love celebrated by Holy Sex is open to life because it rejoices in the creative power of a love so strong it reaches across time and space into future generations. Openness to life enables a couple to say to one another, "We're really not just fooling around here. This is for keeps." Openness to life promises a commitment to a love that will outlive the couple themselves. It's a commitment to a love that will ultimately change the lovers and increase the power of the sexual union to make them want to be better people. As novelist and *New Yorker* editor Peter DeVries once quipped, "The value of marriage is not that adults produce children, but that children produce adults."

This is a sentiment with which the Catholic Church and Pope John Paul II in particular agreed wholeheartedly. A true, unified love is life-giving, not just metaphorically, in the sense of emotionally energizing a couple, but literally, in the procreative sense. Children represent the miraculous unity between a husband and wife like nothing else:

> *Rather than closing them up in themselves, [a couple's unity] opens them up toward new life, toward a new person. As parents, they will be capable of giving life to a being like themselves, not only bone of their bones and flesh of their flesh . . . , but an image and likeness of God — a person.* (John Paul II, Letter to Families)

The idea that children help men and women become better versions of themselves is even evidenced by biology. It is well known that, assuming no physical problems, the chemical changes that occur in a woman during pregnancy and birth make her more nurturing, sensitive, and patient, as well as expanding her biological capacity for generosity. What is less known is that fatherhood actually creates physiological changes in the male that produce similar virtuous effects. A 2006 study in the journal *Nature* revealed that after the birth of offspring, male mammals experienced greater connectivity in the prefrontal cortex, the part of the brain responsible for planning, problem-solving, and managing emotional stress. Likewise, following the birth of offspring, males experience up to a 30 percent reduction in testosterone, as well as elevated levels of cortisol and prolactin, which enable them to be more nurturing and alert. In other words, the presence of children gives *guys* and *girls* the physiological impetus to become *men* and *women.*

Of course, as Mother Teresa was fond of reminding us, Jesus said, "Anyone who welcomes a little child, welcomes me." The couple who truly loves each other and loves Our Lord will welcome the children he wants to give them. Having children is both an incredible privilege and an awesomely exciting responsibility for married couples.

IS EVERY SPERM SACRED?

Of course, the Church's teaching on the creative power of sex is easily misunderstood and misrepresented. Most peoples' education regarding the intricacies of Catholic sexual ethics appears to have begun and ended with Monty Python's *The Meaning of Life*: "Every sperm is sacred, every sperm is great! If a sperm is wasted, God gets quite irate!"

Thanks to our friends at the National Association of Conventional Wisdom on All Things Catholic, everyone knows that the only reason the Church tolerates sex at all is because babies can come of it. Furthermore, when the Church says that every act of intercourse must be open to life, it quite obviously means that unless a couple chances conception every single time they have sex, then sex is bad, and they are bad. And we mean BAAAAAAAAD in capital letters. Surely you got the memo?

Well, if you did, the memo was wrong.

But if Catholics don't think that sex is so vile that only its function as a tool of procreation can redeem it, why do Catholics value the creative power of sex so much? Catholic theologian Janet Smith once wrote that "because God is a lover he is also a creator; his love overflows into the creation of new beings."

God loves loving. Love is what God does best, but a lover isn't much good without a beloved. This is why God seems to be endlessly fascinated with creating new things. It gives him more to love.

G. K. Chesterton once observed that God delights in creation because he loves it so much and loves creating more to love. In his book *Orthodoxy*, Chesterton writes,

> It is possible that God says every morning, "Do it again" to the sun; and every evening "Do it again" to the moon. It may not be automatic necessity that makes the daisies alike; it may be that God makes every daisy separately, but has never gotten tired of making them. It may be that He has the eternal appetite of infancy; for we have sinned and grown old, and our Father is younger than we. The repetition in Nature may not be mere recurrence; it may be a theatrical encore. Heaven may encore the bird who laid an egg. If the human being conceives and brings forth a human child instead of bringing forth a fish, or a bat, or a griffin, the reason may not be that we are fixed in an animal fate without life or

purpose. It may be that our little tragedy has touched the gods, that they admire it from their starry galleries, and that at the end of every human drama man is called again and again before the curtain.

Perhaps this is one of the things Jesus meant when he told us that unless we became like little children we could not enter the kingdom of heaven (Luke 18:15–17). Children never get tired of creating and of repeating a good thing. Neither does God. It is only we sinful, jaded adults who see a field of flowers and think "parking garage" or see a baby and think "second mortgage." By contrast, if a small child — or God — sees the same field of flowers or the same baby, they both think, "Yeah! Do it again!"

Who do you think is living more authentically?

Even though God is completely sufficient on his own, God loves creating, and God especially loves to create people. As the Church tells us, the human being is "the only creature on earth whom God willed for its own sake" (*Gaudium et Spes*). Why? Because we are the only creatures he gets to spend an eternity loving. We are the only earthly beings built to last, so to speak. One can only guess that for God it is a joy beyond words to create creatures whom he can love *eternally*. This same God, who generously longs to share all of his joy with us, gives husbands and wives a taste of the particular joy that is creating and loving the creation by inviting us to bring his children into the world.

AARON AND REBECCA'S STORY

Aaron and Rebecca have been married thirteen years. They have four children and hope to have more.

Rebecca says, "People act shocked when we say we'd like to have more kids. But frankly, I feel sorry for them. I love Aaron, and I love our kids. I just couldn't imagine life without them, and I can't imagine life without the next little person God might want to send our way."

When I ask Aaron how he feels about the idea of having more children, he says, "Rebecca is a great mom and she's a great wife. I think we both work hard to make sure that our marriage and our kids get what they need from us. It takes staying on top of things, but I totally think it's worth it. We don't rush into it. We want to be sure that we can really care for whatever kids we have. Not just financially. I mean, you can always put another potato in the pot, like my grandma used to say. I mean we want to make sure we can really be there for them. When I look at our kids, I think, 'We did that!' and it makes me love Becky even more. It makes me want to do it again."

WE ARE FAM-I-LY! BEING OPEN TO LIFE

In Genesis we are told that man was made in the image and likeness of God (Gen. 1:26). God is a Trinity, and the Trinity represents a loving relationship between persons (Father, Son, and Holy Spirit), whose love creates life and then brings that life back into itself, forming an ever-expanding circle of love and creativity. That's why God created the world, and that's why he redeemed it. He doesn't just create. He wants to bring humanity into himself and make us part of the Trinity through Jesus Christ.

Catholics believe that it is the human family that "images" or, in a sense, puts a human face on how the Trinity works. When a human family is working according to the plan for which God designed it, it too is an ever-expanding circle of love that demands to be expressed through creation, which then demands to be drawn back into the intimate community of persons, and then seeks to create an even bigger love that demands to be expressed through creation. And so on and so on.

There are many people who believe that when children enter the scene, intimacy dies. But this doesn't have to be the case. A study in the *Journal of Infant and Child Development* shows that it is not children that cause marital distress. Rather, it's the strength of the couple's pre-baby relationship that predicts how well parents will be able to protect their intimacy post-baby. These findings were true even for parents who had fussy, temperamental babies. In short, researchers find that children do not kill marriage. Inattention to marriage pre- and post-baby kills marriage. In a later chapter, we'll examine what needs to happen for couples to grow in love *because of* their children rather than in spite of them. For now, we note that when psychologically healthy people invest a reasonable amount of energy in creating an emotionally stable marriage, the advent of children actually causes marital intimacy to increase. On this point, both Catholic teaching and psychological research on the make-up of healthy families are in agreement.

BET YOU DIDN'T KNOW

But openness to life is bigger than mere openness to conception. According to the Church, a couple can be open to life, *even when they have determined not to have more children for a time — or even indefinitely.* How can this be? Well, beyond a willingness to have children, openness to life also requires a couple to be ready to meet the temporal, emotional, and spiritual needs of the children they already have so that those children can be fully functioning, happy, well-adjusted, holy men and women. Furthermore, in a sense that takes on special significance for couples struggling with infertility, openness to life means a couple understands that their passion for one another is bigger than just the two of them and must compel them to bear witness to Christ's passionate love for the world by leading lives of generous service to others or perhaps welcoming the little stranger through adoption.

God gives many benefits to those husbands and wives who celebrate openness to life, *whether or not children are always created as a result.* Each of these benefits manifests another way "the two become one." Practiced according to Church teaching (and not merely according to caricatures of Church teaching), openness to life yields four benefits:

1. Increased passion

2. A new level of communication and prayerful discernment

3. Greater responsiveness to children

4. A truly spiritual sexuality

Increased Passion

All of the pop psych books about "spiritual sex" and "tantric lovemaking" have nothing on the sheer joy, vulnerability, spirituality, and total self-gift that accompanies the phrase "Let's make a baby!" Many books proclaim the virtues of "simultaneous orgasm" and, to be honest, they speak a partial truth. But nothing, absolutely nothing, compares to the profound joy that occurs when *a husband, a wife, and God climax together* — and new life is created. How sad it is that our sexuality has been so perverted by the pagans and misrepresented by the media that a statement such as the one I just made might actually be shocking to many of you reading this book. But the fact remains, sex is a good. *God gave sex to the godly.* The pagans stole it from us when we weren't looking, and it's time we take it back. Through the procreative work of marriage, God gives us the grace to do just that. He empowers us to experience real love, which is a life-giving love.

It would be ridiculous to suggest that openness to life is a virtue that could exist without a focus on children, but even when *conception* is not the *immediate* focus — either because of infertility or because of the decision to postpone a pregnancy through licit means (Natural Family Planning) and for good reasons — openness to life can bring great blessings to the couple's sexual relationship by communicating a total acceptance of one's partner.

All of us want to be loved totally. Every single one of us wants to be loved completely. We long to give all of ourselves to another and have every bit of ourselves received joyfully and openly in return. When a couple is closed to life — whether through contraception, sterilization, or simply by means of a cold, closed heart — the couple accepts only the parts of each other that make them feel good and rejects all the parts of each other that promise the commitment and responsibility of real love.

PETER AND LYNNETTE'S STORY

Peter and Lynnette contacted me for counseling to address an unsatisfying sexual relationship. Peter was frustrated by the infrequency of intercourse and his wife's poor response to his attempts to please her. Lynnette complained of a profoundly decreased libido and painful intercourse. Consultations with her gynecologist revealed no medical problems, and the attempts to practice vaginal dilation exercises (inserting different sized vaginal dilators to relax and stretch the vaginal walls prescribed by the physician) and utilize lubricants failed to produce the desired results.

Over the course of several sessions, Lynnette confessed that she was terrified that Peter would leave her if they got pregnant. "I know he loves me. But when we talk about having a child, he gets so angry and defensive. He's adamant. He gets angry if I just bring it up. He just totally shuts down and refuses to talk to me at all. If something happened and I got pregnant, I don't think he would have anything to do with me. I take birth control, but I know people who've gotten pregnant anyway. I'm terrified of what he'd do if I got pregnant."

The couple was weighed down under a mountain of debt due to Peter's graduate school loans, and he was determined to get their finances under control before they had a child. Lynnette agreed that it would not necessarily be prudent to conceive at the time, but the intensity of Peter's refusal to even talk about having children — whether in the immediate or distant future — conveyed a deep sense of rejection to Lynnette. She became phobic of sex as a means of preserving their relationship. Her body responded to Peter's rejection of her fertility with a severely retarded libido and a condition called vaginismus, the involuntary contracting of the vaginal walls combined with a lack of lubrication that at best makes sex painful and, at worst, can prevent penetration altogether.

Over the course of their therapy, the couple learned to open up the discussion about having children. Peter reassured Lynnette that his intensity about not having a child right now did not mean that he was not desirous of children in the future, and that even if they were to get pregnant he would never leave her. Together, they made two financial plans. First, they made a budget to describe how they would live if they did conceive before the debt was paid. It would be tight, but Peter understood that he was being more fearful about their financial situation than he needed to be. He realized that a baby, should one be born even under their present financial circumstances, would hardly destroy them. This simple action, combined with a little reality check, helped both Peter and Lynnette contend realistically with the fact that sex causes babies, sometimes when you least expect it.

Second, they established a concrete budget that would allow them to pay off their debt and a realistic timeframe for when they would seriously and intentionally begin pursuing parenthood. These activities, combined with some basic communication and relationship-building exercises, brought about a dramatic change in the couples' lovemaking. Lynnette could experience her love and passion for Peter unencumbered by the fear of abandonment caused by Peter's rejection of the creative aspects of their love.

Some readers might object to this case study by saying that Lynnette's sexual problems were the result of repressed Catholic guilt, but Peter and Lynnette were raised in minimally Protestant homes and were unchurched at the time of their meetings with me. There was no religious baggage weighing down their sexuality. The only thing holding Lynnette back from real passion was the knowledge that Peter simply didn't want all of her; that his love and desire for her were limited solely to the parts of her that could make *him* feel good, which she correctly and viscerally understood was really not much of a love at all. Not all couples experience the kind of dramatic problems Peter and Lynnette did, but closing sex off to the possibility of new life drains a significant portion of the meaningfulness and significance out of the sexual relationship and increases the risk that the couple will view sex as merely recreation, leading them to take it, and each other, for granted. Even if a couple has decided that they have legitimate reasons to postpone a pregnancy, keeping the option open for a future date and continuing to discuss the possibility of more children consistently reminds couples that as far as sex is concerned, there is more than play at stake. There is mystery. There is power. There is joy in the possibility of new life for the couple and for the world.

Peter and Lynnette's marital problems and recovery offers us a fascinating look at how openness to life *as a virtue* enables a couple to actualize their passion for one another even in cases where conception isn't the immediate goal. Again, openness to life does require and assume an openness to conception, but openness to conception is not the sole expression of an openness to life.

Deeper Communication

The second benefit that openness to life brings to a couple is that it leads to a new level of communication and increases their capacity for mutual prayer and discernment.

Even when a couple has valid reasons for delaying or postponing pregnancy, the joy of continuing to be open to life brings a more profound dimension to lovemaking. This is possible because of the benefits of Natural Family Planning (NFP) that extend beyond its ability to help couples either achieve or avoid pregnancy.

We will discuss common questions about NFP in chapter 10, but for now, it is sufficient to look at the practical wisdom behind the Church's endorsement of NFP that extends beyond the moral arguments. NFP and contraception exemplify radically different mind-sets about sexuality.

On the one hand, contraception:

- is almost always one spouse's responsibility (usually, the woman's)

- treats pregnancy as a disease that should be prevented

- often has harmful side effects (as I advise throughout this book, read the inserts for your chemical contraception of choice)

- is prone to failure (carrying with it spousal condemnation along with pregnancy)

- makes sex habitual rather than special, presenting physical barriers to complete unity

- sends the message that you don't want all of your mate (just the parts that give you pleasure)

- can make conceiving a baby and sustaining a pregnancy very difficult even after you stop using it.

This last point is especially true with regard to chemical contraception, which can prevent a woman from conceiving months after she stops taking it, and even if she does become pregnant it can increase the risk of miscarriage, again for months after she stops taking it.

On the other hand, NFP:

* is the shared responsibility of a husband and wife

* facilitates communication between them about each others' bodies

* requires a husband and wife to continually talk and pray about their priorities and keeps in play discussions about becoming or being parents

* is completely natural with no side effects

* has been found again and again (particularly the Creighton model) to be over 99 percent effective (a 2007 study of sixteen hundred women by the University of Heidelberg published in *Human Reproduction Today* found NFP to be as effective as the Pill in preventing pregnancy)

* keeps lovemaking fresh and exciting by building in little breaks for the couple to work on their overall marriage

* requires the couple to focus on relationship and romance rather than just habitual sex

* can even be an extraordinarily useful tool for helping couples intentionally conceive. (In fact, ob/gyns use modified forms of NFP as a first-line treatment of infertility.)

Couples who practice NFP are empowered to seek God's will for their lives in a way no contracepting couple ever can. They are challenged to communicate and share on an intimate, personal, and physical level that makes many contracepting couples uncomfortable. NFP couples practice "sex for real," and this kind of sex has it all over every other kind there is.

In his *Letter to Families*, Pope John Paul II noted that unlike what often happens with contracepting couples, the couple who works together to prayerfully discern *each month* whether or not God is calling them to have a child accepts that "both are responsible for their potential and later actual fatherhood and motherhood. The husband cannot fail to acknowledge and accept the result of a decision that has also been his own. He cannot hide behind such expressions as: 'I don't know,' 'I didn't want it,' or 'You're the one who wanted it.'"

The sexuality that NFP empowers a couple to give to one another is beautiful, creative, passionate, intentional, responsible, mutually caring, mutually consented to, and prayerfully discerned. Because NFP challenges couples to achieve such a high level of communication, prayer, and co-operation, it is little wonder that NFP couples have a significantly lower divorce rate than other couples. Some studies report that the divorce rate for NFP couples is only 5 percent compared to 50 percent in the general population. Although more research needs to be done to verify these dramatic findings, even if the divorce rate for NFP couples was five times what this study claimed, it would still be half the divorce rate for contracepting couples. Clearly, something is going on here.

The case of Max and Wendy illustrates the power of the virtue of openness to life to transform a couple's communication and prayer life.

MAX AND WENDY'S STORY

Max and Wendy have been married fifteen years and have four children. In the early years of their marriage, they didn't believe that NFP was really effective. Says Max, "We believed the old joke that said, 'What do you call a couple that uses NFP? Parents.'"

Still, after three years on the Pill, the couple found that they were having a hard time conceiving their first child. Their physician explained that the effects of the Pill are not immediately reversible in all women, and that it can take several cycles before the Pill can completely wash out of a woman's body. The doctor advised them to keep trying.

After several months, the couple was no closer to conceiving when a friend told Wendy how some of the signs couples record when doing NFP can be used to help diagnose problems achieving pregnancy,

Wendy says, "I thought it had to be some kind of voodoo, but by then I was ready for voodoo or anything else anyone was willing to suggest."

The couple learned the Symptothermal Method of NFP, which involves temperature checks and learning about other bodily cues. Within two cycles, Wendy discovered that her signs were consistent with impaired thyroid function. Max and Wendy consulted with a nutritionist recommended by their NFP trainers and were able to begin nutritional supplements that corrected the imbalance naturally. Two months later, Wendy's cycles displayed a normal pattern. A month later, Wendy and Max were pregnant.

Max adds, "We just figured that if NFP could tell us so much about Wendy's body that we could use it to get pregnant, we could use it the other way too." (Note: to avoid pregnancy, NFP users abstain from sex for about seven to ten days, depending upon the length of the fertile phase of the woman's cycle.) Max and Wendy went on to have three more children spaced about three years apart using the method. Beyond the direct benefits to their fertility, Max and Wendy reported being surprised by other advantages.

As Wendy explains, "Our teaching couple told us that NFP would help with our communication and prayer lives, but we didn't really buy that at the time. We just wanted to have a baby. But once we started using NFP to space our kids, Max and I started talking a lot more about whether any given month it was time to have another child or not. We'd regularly weigh the pros and cons of having more kids. We'd pray about all that stuff, and we never really prayed together before that. Because the question was always out there, we talked a lot more about our dreams, and where we thought we were going as a couple and a family. We didn't do that nearly the same way before we were using NFP."

Max says, "Sometimes taking time off from sex can feel a little frustrating, but Wendy and I tried really hard to connect by taking the time to talk and pray together. It was different at first. Before we didn't talk as much. We'd be tired, and so we'd just use sex to keep us together. Not that I minded at the time, of course, but now I see how much closer we are. Our marriage is tons better because we've had to think about it more. NFP made us more intentional about sex, too. We don't take it for granted. Although it's spaced out a little *differently, we make love as often as we used to. Probably more. And it's a lot better, I think, because we're closer all around."*

Wendy adds, *"We really do love each other more now, and I think that has everything to do with the changes NFP brought to our marriage. Sex is better because we're better people. Better friends."*

Even when a couple is taking some time off from conception, the virtue of openness to life always helps to remind the couple that sex is about more than just fun. It's *always* about love *and life too*. The virtue of openness to life challenges a couple to discuss and pray each month about their priorities and discern whether this month is time to work harder on caring for each other and the children they already have, or if this month is time to try to add another little member to their community of love. Openness to life means that the couple is always open to whatever new possibilities God has in store for them, and that openness to grace has direct benefits to the couple's overall intimacy, not just their sexual intimacy.

Parenthood, Responsibly

Of course, the true joy of Catholic procreation (and this is the part you'll never hear about in the media) is that it doesn't stop at conception. When Catholics say "yes" to the gift of a child, the Church teaches that we must also be in a position to say "yes" to the forming of that child's body, mind, and soul. This is what the Catholic Church calls "integral procreation." Catholics believe that procreation is a continuous event that extends from the moment of conception to the time our children are able to stand on their own two feet before God. Procreation is the act by which Christians co-operate with God to form minds and souls, not just bodies. Or, as John Paul II puts it in his *Letter to Families*, "Fatherhood and motherhood represent a responsibility which is not simply physical but spiritual in nature."

The National Association for Conventional Wisdom on All Things Catholic would have you believe that the "Catholic thing to do" is to have as many children as you can in as short a time as possible, regardless of whether you can remember their names, much less form them as persons. Nothing could be further from the truth, and if any parents approach childbearing in this manner, they do it with the express disapproval of Catholic teaching. As Dr. Janet Smith, author of *Contraception, Why Not?* asserts, "The Church does not teach that women are obliged to have as many children as their bodies can bear."

Pope John Paul II, in his July 1994 Angelus address, stated:

> *Unfortunately, Catholic thought is often misunderstood on this point, as if the Church supported an ideology of fertility at all costs, urging married couples to procreate indiscriminately and without thought for the future. But one need only study the pronouncements of the Magisterium to know that this is not so. Truly, in begetting life the spouses fulfill one of the highest dimensions of their calling: they are God's co-workers. Precisely for this reason they must have an extremely responsible attitude. In deciding whether or not to have a child, they must not be motivated by selfishness or carelessness, but by a prudent, conscious generosity that weighs the possibilities and circumstances, and especially gives priority to the welfare of the unborn child. Therefore, when there is a reason not to procreate, this choice is permissible and may even be necessary.*

The Church has always taught that it is not sufficient to have a passel of children. Rather, parents' primary obligation is to have only as many children as they believe they can *educate and form* into healthy, loving, godly persons. As it says in Scripture: "Desire not a brood of worthless children, nor rejoice in wicked offspring. Many though they be, exult not in them if they have not the fear of the Lord. Count not on their length of life, have no hope for their future. For one [child] can be better than a thousand; rather die childless than have godless children" (Sir. 16:1–3).

Of course children are a blessing, and the Church encourages couples to have as many children as they can properly form, which is probably more than most people have. But the point of having children, for the Catholic, is not accumulating numbers and racking up points in some holiness-by-the-numbers spiritual-pyramid scheme. Rather, the point of procreation is to bring as many new members into God's Kingdom as parents can properly form to love God and know God's love for them.

Considering the popular perception that Catholics are obliged by "official Church teaching" to have a fetish for indiscriminate procreation, it's ironic that the above verse was taken from Sirach, a book found only in the Bibles of Catholic and Orthodox Christians. The book of Sirach was part of the canon of Scripture for all Christians for over a millennium and a half, until it was removed in the 1500s by Protestant reformers. Interestingly, this is one of the few verses of Scripture that does not consider children an automatic blessing. Without this Scripture passage, responsible parenthood as a *biblical* teaching would most likely not be possible. My point, of course, is that indiscriminate procreation, rather than being a Catholic concept, would really be the product of a literal reading of the *Protestant* Scriptures. This point is not just theoretical — it's evidenced by the Protestant "Quiverful Movement" (see *www.quiverful.com*). Adherents of the Quiverful Movement (see Ps. 127:3–5) argue that even Natural Family Planning is contrary to the Scriptures and that the *only* biblical option for Christian couples is to have sex and see what happens. By including and retaining Sirach in its Bible, the Catholic Church also asserts responsible, intentional parenthood from its very foundations.

Even when couples experience infertility, retaining the generous heart of service that exists at the core of the virtue of openness to life can lead to great blessings. In the words of St. Josemaría Escrivá, the founder of Opus Dei:

> God in His providence has two ways of blessing marriages: one by giving them children; and the other, sometimes, because he loves them so much, by not giving them children. I don't know which is the better blessing. In any event, let one accept his own.

According to Catholic theologian Scott Hahn, in *Ordinary Work, Extraordinary Grace*, St. Josemaría Escrivá encouraged those couples who were struggling with infertility to practice openness to life in a broader sense. "St. Josemaría taught them to love one another dearly and to spend their love lavishly on the people around them — to give more of their time to [ministry work] and service among friends.... Thus their lives, like the lives of parents, will be full."

Whether or not couples are able to have children and whether or not couples are actively pursuing conception in a given month, the virtue of openness to life reminds couples that the secret to happiness cannot be found in Wallerstein's Romantic Anti-Marriage, which we discussed earlier, but rather can be found only by celebrating a love that is generative.

The Church recognizes that the desire for more children can become so intoxicating that some Christians may be tempted to pursue that joy as an end in itself, without regard to their responsibility for properly nourishing the bodies, minds, and souls of children entrusted to their care. To counter this potentially harmful tendency, the Church teaches responsible parenthood (see *Humanae Vitae, Familiaris Consortio*). That is, in discerning God's will for the size of our families, we are obliged to consider the resources (or lack thereof) God has given us to provide for the physical, emotional, and spiritual needs of a child. The following passage from the adult catechism, *The Teaching of Christ*, and from the Vatican II document *Gaudium et Spes* (The Church in the Modern World) offers an excellent summary of this teaching.

> *For while a child is a great blessing, it is sometimes very important for parents to give careful thought to the size of their families. Husband and wife "will thoughtfully take into account both their own welfare and that of their children, those already born and those which may be foreseen. For this accounting they will reckon with both the material and the spiritual conditions of the times as well as their state of life. Finally, they will consult the interests of the family group, of temporal society, and of the Church herself. The parents themselves should ultimately make this judgment, in the sight of God" (GS, 50).*

In short, responsible parenthood makes parents more responsive to God's will for their lives, to the children they already have, and to their obligation to share the love Christ gives to the couple through meaningful and generative service to the world at large.

Spiritual Sexuality — From Slavery to Freedom

The man who abstains from bodily pleasures and delights in this very fact is temperate, while the man who is annoyed at it is self-indulgent.

(Aristotle, 366 B.C., *Nicomachean Ethics*)

In my counseling practice, I've never met anyone who likes himself *because* he drinks too much, eats too much, plays too much, sleeps too much, or otherwise abuses himself. Caving in to every whim of our bodies is one of the quickest ways to destroy self-esteem. That's why people who eat, drink, play, and sleep in moderation are happier and healthier than people who don't do enough of those things, or do them too much. The same is true about sex.

The neuroendocrine system of the brain — part of the lower brain, which humans share with other animals — is responsible for anger, hunger, and sex drives. It is curious that almost every person, whether a counseling professional, clergy, or layperson, agrees that gaining control over one's anger and hunger drives makes us more human, indeed even heroically so, while seeking to gain mastery over one's sex drive — so that one can choose the best way and the best time to give oneself to another — makes us prudes. This is absurd from both logical and biological points of view, as Aristotle noted almost four hundred years before anyone ever even heard of "Catholic guilt."

I hardly think that any sane person would argue the point that there are about a million ways we can use our sexuality to abuse ourselves and others. Most commonly, we treat our sexuality like it was a street drug we take to make us happy. Or we use it to inflate a pathetic self-image ("Hey! I can't be all bad. I got some!"). Not only does this reduce a person to his or her least common denominator (even insects "get some," after all); it hurts others because it turns them into things to be used (or things to be resented when they refuse to be used).

164

Any abuse of self or others decreases our chances of "being happy with him in heaven." Because of this, husbands and wives are encouraged by the Church to make use of periodic abstinence (as practiced in Natural Family Planning) as a *spiritual exercise* to help each other master, purify, and perfect their sexuality. By the way, this is not only a Catholic phenomenon. Hinduism, Buddhism, and several popular Eastern texts on spiritual sexuality all speak of the benefits of sexual abstinence in various forms. In fact, I believe virtually every major spiritual system on earth (except, of course, American pop-psych and the high priests of pop-spirituality at NACWATC) values some form of abstinence as a means of purifying both sexuality and the human person.

Developing control over the sexual impulse enables us to give ourselves at the right time, to the right person, and in the right manner. Rather than making sex a mechanical, animalistic bodily function, self-control is what lies at the heart of becoming an Infallible Lover because one primary requirement of Infallible Loving is that I must be free. What does that mean?

The secular world thinks that freedom means "being able to do whatever I feel like doing whenever I feel like doing it." But that isn't freedom. That's merely slavery to my emotions. Is it freedom to have to give vent to every angry thought that pops into my head? Is it freedom to feel that I must eat whenever and whatever my feelings tell me I want to eat? Is it freedom to insist on my right to have sex any way I want, with whomever I want, whenever I want? No. If I want to be truly free, I must be able to resist the emotional impulses that attempt to order me to act in a manner contrary to my well-being and the well-being of those I love. If I am compelled by my sexual drive to demand sex from my wife whenever I want it, regardless of her feelings, and then pout if she doesn't give in to me, am I truly free to love her as she deserves to be loved?

I'd say the answer is no. I can love my wife only if I have enough control over myself to consider what she wants and needs from me first and make sure that I am meeting my relationship needs in a manner that is respectful of hers. That kind of authentic, intentional, respectful love — what we are calling "Infallible Love" — takes mindfulness and effort.

Incidentally, you will recall from our earlier discussions that what I've been talking about is the real definition of the virtue known as "chastity." Most people think that chastity simply means, "White knuckle your way through sexual abstinence until you get married, then do whatever you want." But that isn't it at all. Rather, chastity refers to the ability to love well and properly. As the *Encyclopedia of Catholic Doctrine* puts it:

> *Chastity is the virtue that enables one to use one's sexual powers properly. The chaste person is in control of his or her sexual desires rather than being controlled by them. Chastity frees one from being dominated by one's sexual passions. Necessary for both the married and unmarried, chastity is rooted in deep respect for the other person, who should never be used as a means to satisfy one's sexual desires. The power of sexuality allows one to make a gift of oneself to another. Again, chastity is the virtue that allows one to make a proper use of that power.*

It is chastity — the ability to choose the best way, time, and place to give myself to my spouse — that makes it possible to consider sex as a sanctifying, spiritual enterprise. Without the freedom to choose the best way to make a gift of yourself to your beloved, sex is merely an itch to be scratched. There is nothing holy about that.

When a couple approaches each other with true love and the kind of respect that works hard to avoid the temptation to use each other as a means to an end, it's possible to celebrate Holy Sex, a truly spiritual sexuality that increases a couple's passion for one another, views lovemaking as an invitation to achieve a new level of communication and prayerful discernment, makes one more responsive to the needs of others (especially children), and connects the lovers to God's own love.

PART THREE

The School of Love

P ope John Paul II often referred to families as "schools of love." Having explored the differences between Holy Sex and eroticism and discovered the five amazing powers of Holy Sex, in Part Three we will examine some simple ways couples can turn their marriages into schools of love where they learn the steps of Infallible Loving and celebrate the fullness of all Five Powers of Holy Sex.

10 QUESTIONS ABOUT NATURAL FAMILY PLANNING

[The Church is not] inconsistent when she considers it lawful for married people to take advantage of the infertile period but condemns as always unlawful the use of means which directly prevent conception, even when the reasons given for the latter practice may appear to be upright and serious. In reality, these two cases are completely different. In the former the married couple rightly use a faculty provided them by nature. In the latter they obstruct the natural development of the generative process. It cannot be denied that in each case the married couple, for acceptable reasons, are both perfectly clear in their intention to avoid children and wish to make sure that none will result. But it is equally true that it is exclusively in the former case that husband and wife are ready to abstain from intercourse during the fertile period as often as for reasonable motives the birth of another child is not desirable. And when the infertile period recurs, they use their married intimacy to express their mutual love and safeguard their fidelity toward one another. In doing this they certainly give proof of a true and authentic love.

— Pope Paul VI, *Humanae Vitae*

I have briefly touched on the issue of Natural Family Planning (NFP) in several other sections of this book. Now we're bringing it all together. In this chapter, after focusing on some important points that have not yet been covered elsewhere, I'll respond to common questions and objections to NFP.

NFP is a means of both achieving and postponing pregnancy. Thanks to the fine people at the National Association for Conventional Wisdom on All Things Catholic (NACWATC), many believe that the Church rejects contraception because it gives couples the power to choose whether or not to have another child. This view, as the epigraph from *Humanae Vitae* that began this chapter shows, is ignorant and wrong.

The sin of contraception is that it unnaturally rips apart the natural order that God created in a woman's cycle. It treats fertility as a disease and children as an unwelcome by-product of sex. It allows men to further victimize women and view them as sexual objects instead of persons and partners. As Pope Paul VI put it in *Humanae Vitae*:

> *Reflect on the consequences of methods and plans for artificial birth control. Let them first consider how easily this course of action could open wide the way for marital infidelity and a general lowering of moral standards. . . . Another effect that gives cause for alarm is that a man who grows accustomed to the use of contraceptive methods may forget the reverence due to a woman, and, disregarding her physical and emotional equilibrium, reduce her to being a mere instrument for the satisfaction of his own desires, no longer considering her as his partner whom he should surround with care and affection.*

If you don't want to hear from a Catholic leader, how about a Hindu? Here's Mahatma Gandhi on the same point.

> *It is an insult to the fair sex to put up her case in support of birth-control by artificial methods. As it is, man has sufficiently degraded her for his lust and artificial methods . . . will still further degrade her. I urge advocates of artificial methods to consider the consequences. . . . Birth control to me is a dismal abyss.*

I referred above to the "sin" of contraception. People get squeamish around the word "sin." I want to take a moment to define the term. Despite conventional wisdom, something is *not* sinful because it is cooked up by demons who like to hang out in the back alley behind the home office of Evil Super-Villains-R-Us. Rather, something is sinful for three reasons:

1. It represents settling for less than God wants to give us.

2. It violates the natural order God created in the world, which can lead to the breakdown of the human person and his or her physical, psychological, moral, and spiritual well-being.

3. It treats people as things.

Contraception is sinful because — as you discovered in our look at the Fifth Power of Holy Sex — it causes the spouses to say, "I don't want all of you. Please check your fertility at the door. I don't want to be *that* committed, *that* responsible, *that* accountable to you. Just give me the parts of you that make me feel good."

Second, contraception is sinful because it rips apart the natural order God created, jeopardizing a woman's health (read the inserts that accompany hormonal contraceptives), and treats babies as hostile invaders (leading to abortion's status — enshrined by the U.S. Supreme Court — as a necessary means of dealing with failed contraception). Believe it or not, hormonal contraception also spoils the environment. Regarding the last point, in 2006 the British Environmental Agency released a report indicating that fully a third of the male fish living near water treatment plants in the U.K. are changing sex and producing eggs because of the presence of contraceptive hormones present in the rivers (they are not eliminated by water treatment). The same report found that elevated contraceptive hormones in the water supply has caused human male sperm count to fall by 30 percent in thirteen years in Britain, leading to one-in-six couples struggling with infertility. If chemical companies were dumping pesticides in the water that had this effect on wildlife, the public would be screaming for justice, but when it comes to the human pesticide that is contraception, very few bat an eye. We've been too brainwashed.

Third, contraception is sinful because it treats the people who are making love as mere instruments of giving and receiving pleasure. In other words, people who use contraception are not being lovers to each other. They are simply using their bodies as elaborate sex toys, designed solely for the purpose of giving and receiving pleasure.

I have outlined other problems with contraception previously in this book. To briefly recap, contraception tends to become the "woman's responsibility," leading to resentment in the relationship and possibly charges of irresponsibility by the husband in the event of contraception failure and pregnancy. If nonchemical, barrier methods of contraception are used, these violate the unity of the couple and may actually impair the physiological bonding process. Further, contraception continues to affect a couple's ability to conceive and sustain pregnancy for months after the couple stops using it. Also, chemical contraception *can cause abortion* because, when it fails to prevent ovulation, it prevents a fertilized egg from implanting in the uterus. Physicians often attempt to deny the abortifacient properties of chemical contraception by saying that life does not begin until implantation, and since chemical contraception prevents implantation, then there's no abortion. But this is dishonest. Implantation does not define human life. Fertilization does. Everything the person needs to be a human being — all the genetic coding that will be with them for life — is present at fertilization. Because of this, the Pill kills.

For all these reasons and more, the Church proclaims that contraception is bad for the soul, bad for women's health, bad for babies, bad for relationships, and bad for the environment. NFP, in all its many forms, suffers from none of these problems. It's a reliable, healthy, ecological means of both achieving and postponing pregnancy. It's beneficial to relationships because it challenges couples to grow in all the virtues that lead to intimacy and a healthy sexuality. As research published in both the *International Review of Natural Family Planning* and the *Linacre Quarterly* has shown, couples who use NFP have significantly lower rates of divorce than couples who contracept. Further (for reasons discussed earlier), NFP causes a couple to be open to life even when they're actively working to postpone pregnancy. It is the shared responsibility of husband and wife.

Finally, NFP enables couples to be better sexual partners to one another because they know each other's bodies better. For instance, a woman's body changes dramatically based upon which phase of her monthly cycle she is in. During the phase of her cycle when she is fertile, her cervix is higher up, and she experiences greater degrees of lubrication, making sexual positions that allow deeper penetration and vigorous lovemaking more easily possible. In the times of the month when she is infertile, her cervix is lower and she experiences less lubrication, requiring her lover to spend more time on foreplay to increase lubrication and to take time in lovemaking before moving to positions that allow for deeper penetration. Couples who use NFP are less likely to experience frustrations related to sexual communication or performance because the man knows intimately how his wife's body works. This level of intimate understanding enables couples to communicate more easily about the best way to please each other.

In short, NFP is permitted by the Church and is not sinful, not because it has anything to do with the conscious choice to have or not have children, but because it respects the natural order God created a woman's cycle to operate by and is therefore good for her soul, good for her health, good for babies, good for relationships, and good for the environment. Where contraception is a negative force, NFP — whether used to conceive or avoid conception — is a positive force for good between the couple and for the world.

SPICE-ING IT UP: SEXUAL INTIMACY

Some couples report that NFP is too frustrating because it requires a couple to abstain for a period of time in the months when they are trying to avoid conception. This is usually about a week to ten days, although this time can vary depending upon the particulars of the woman's cycle and the expertise of the couple. We will deal with the issue of sexual frustration in relation to NFP in chapter 15.

Other couples, however, report that NFP is a blessing to their sexual relationship and passion. As a clinician who has encountered or worked with thousands of NFP-using couples through my radio program and tele-counseling practice, I have a unique window for viewing the blessing that NFP can be to couples.

Done properly, and with the right understanding, NFP can be a kind of master class in sexuality, a real education in Infallible Loving, because it employs a concept known as SPICE. SPICE (an acronym for Spiritual, Physical, Intellectual, Creative, and Emotional) is best understood as the conscious effort a couple makes to enflame their desire for one another and enhance their intimacy by taking short breaks (about a week or so) from genital intercourse while at the same time intensifying the amount of nongenital physical contact (kissing, cuddling, "making out" without going all the way, etc.) and other expressions of affection (such as praying together, making daily time to talk, challenging each other to learn something new together, playing together, making time to share their hopes and dreams).

For example, if you and your mate were trying to avoid pregnancy in a given month and the fertile phase of the wife's cycle lasted ten days, then on each of those ten days you would make a date with your partner to do any or all of the following: cuddle together, make out without going all the way, play a game, work on a project, go out together, and so on. On the tenth day, while you were cuddling, you might tell each other all the pleasures that you have in store for each other on the following evening. On the eleventh day and thereafter you and your mate break your fast, permitting yourselves to feast on the banquet of love you have been planning for days.

Obviously, SPICE can be a powerful expression of marital love. It benefits the couple in four major ways. First, it helps them remember the many other ways a couple needs to say "I love you" besides through sexual intercourse. Lovemaking is wonderful, but many couples come to rely on it exclusively as their way of demonstrating affection, forgetting that serving each other throughout the day, cuddling, and other expressions of love can be just as important and just as sweet.

Second, when Infallible Lovers both willingly and cheerfully surrender their sexual claims to one another — even if only for a short period of time each month — it allows them to see that, more than mere gratification, the *relationship* is the essential center of their sexuality. By enhancing respect for each partner and for the strength of the marriage, the couple leaves little room for either mate to ever, even fleetingly, feel used or taken for granted.

Third, suspending lovemaking for a time requires the couple to communicate and solve conflicts rather than merely "sexing" their way through problems, as all couples are wont to do at one time or another (especially the Positive Materialists). Sex therapists and marriage counselors are well aware of this phenomenon and regularly prescribe some form of creative abstinence (called sensate focus) to help clients recalibrate their relationships.

Finally, and most importantly, periodic abstinence has the potential to raise lovemaking to a high art form and means to actualization. Think about it. Great painters are celebrated as much for their "use of space" as they are for their ability to fill up a canvas with meaningful shapes, colors, and images. Great composers are praised equally for their use of sound and their use of silence to evoke certain moods through their music. In the same way, truly great lovers know how to use both "tension" and "release" to experience the full force of a passion that is uniquely spiritual, uniquely sensual, and uniquely theirs.

Creative abstinence and concepts related to SPICE have been praised in periodicals as diverse as the pop-culture chronicler *Notorious* and the mainstream women's magazine *Redbook*. The author Thomas Moore devotes a whole section of his book *The Soul of Sex* to "The Joy of Celibacy" in marriage. And little wonder. Besides raising lovemaking to a high art form, creative abstinence and SPICE are means to actualization because they allow you to practice your virtues — one set at a time. When you both are making love, you can become more generous, passionate, open, vulnerable, expressive, and so on, and when you are not making love you can become more temperate, patient, self-controlled, sensitive, wise, caring, serving, and so on. Yes, of course, you can develop all of your virtues even if you don't practice SPICE, but taking a short "time-out" from lovemaking each month allows you to focus on certain qualities *exclusively*, like the sculptor who says, "Today I am going to concentrate intimately on the details of my model's hands." It is this sense of detail — craftsmanship, if you will — that allows Infallible Lovers to become masters of the sexual arts, indeed, masters of the art of life in general.

This is so because Infallible Lovers don't think of lovemaking as "the thing we do when we're naked," but rather, "the way we celebrate our relationship all day long." Holy Sex, as I have argued before in this book, is as much social intercourse as it is sexual intercourse. Infallible Lovers know how to feel as close to each other painting a room together as they do lying in each other's arms. That doesn't mean Holy Sex is no more exciting than watching paint dry! It means that every time Infallible Lovers work side-by-side, they experience an intense sexual charge between them. While lovemaking is the most exalted form of communicating their love for each other, Infallible Lovers know that the "words" their bodies speak to one another in lovemaking will be empty and meaningless unless they refer back to the mutual service, outstanding rapport, and intense desire they share all day long. While lesser lovers roll over in bed and say, out-of-the-blue, "You wanna do it?" Infallible Lovers have been engaging in extended foreplay all day through "social intercourse," and frequent, intense, passionate, spiritual lovemaking is the spontaneous, logical result.

A PATH TO PERSONAL AND SPIRITUAL GROWTH

Another way NFP benefits the sexual relationship is by serving as an invitation to explore the deeper meanings of sex. I have suggested throughout this book that Holy Sex is a means of personal, relational, and spiritual growth. If this is true — and it is — then NFP is a catalyst that empowers that growth, propelling couples toward perfection in authentic love.

When we examined the creative power of Holy Sex (the Fifth Power), we discussed the concept of responsible parenthood, which is really the call to balance two sets of virtues. On the one hand, couples are called to exercise the virtue of being open to life. Openness to life challenges couples to exercise virtues like trust in God's providence, a generosity rooted in generativity, and a further identification with the paternity of God. On the other hand, practicing this openness to life responsibly challenges us to live out another, related, but complementary set of virtues including self-control, generosity rooted in intentional loving, chastity, prudence, and temperance. NFP, because it invites the couple to pray, communicate, and discern where God is leading their relationship from month to month, empowers couples to balance and expand their capacity to exhibit both sets of virtues. In this way, NFP challenges couples to "be perfect as the Heavenly Father is perfect (Matt. 5:48)," that is, perfect in love.

The Church tells us that when couples respond to this challenge, they begin to look more and more like the Trinity, in whose image and likeness the human family is made. Once again, we see an example of how Christian eros enables the lovers to rise in ecstasy toward the Divine.

Having offered a basic overview of NFP, I would like to spend the next few pages responding to common questions and objections about NFP and family planning. The following is not intended to be an exhaustive list, but given my experience with the questions on the minds of many couples, I think it will be thorough enough to address the main points.

NFP AND FERTILITY: FREQUENTLY ASKED QUESTIONS

"How does it work?"

First, a cautionary warning. *Do not use the information contained in this section to attempt NFP!* I do not intend this section to be, in any way, viewed as adequate instruction on how to use NFP. Couples interested in Natural Family Planning should contact their local diocesan Family Life Office or Catholic hospital, or make use of the resources listed at the end of this chapter (p. 189). The following serves merely as the most basic outline.

A woman's cycle is divided into three phases. Phase I corresponds with the woman's period and the time immediately following (whether or not the menstrual flow continues). Phase II is the fertile phase of her cycle, when she can conceive. During Phase II, the woman's cervix is soft, high, open, and wet, her cervical mucus is wet and runny (like a runny nose), and her basal body temperature rises noticeably. (Note: basal temperature is measured with a special, very sensitive, basal temperature thermometer. You cannot use the same thermometer you use when checking for fevers.) During Phase III of her cycle, the infertile phase, which begins a few days after ovulation, her cervix lowers and becomes harder and comparatively drier. Her cervical mucus dries up (more like a stuffy nose), and her basal body temperature drops.

Each woman's signs are unique, but once a couple is able to recognize the signs consistent with each stage of their own particular cycle, the couple can predict with over 99 percent accuracy whether they are fertile or infertile.

"Is NFP 'rhythm'?"

No! NFP is not rhythm and has not been "rhythm" since condoms were made of sheep intestines. So knock it off already with the "rhythm" garbage, or I will be forced to come to your house and beat you up for being so stupid. (Deep breaths, deep breaths. Ahhh. I feel better now.)

That said, even Calendar Rhythm (a.k.a., the "Standard Days Method"), which assumes a constant number of days between each phase for each month, has been shown to be over 95 percent effective in avoiding pregnancy, according to the Georgetown University Institute for Reproductive Health. Some people still practice this method of family planning, although it is not the most reliable form available.

In contrast to the Standard Days Method, modern NFP is a highly sophisticated, easy-to-use, scientific method for achieving or avoiding pregnancy.

"Is there more than one way to do NFP?"

Yes. There are many methods of doing NFP, all of which help couples evaluate physical signs to determine which phase of her cycle a woman is in (e.g., cervical mucus signs, cervical position, basal temperature, hormonal levels). All of the following methods have been consistently shown to be over 99 percent effective — as effective as chemical contraception without the physical, relational, and environmental side effects.

- *The Symptothermal Method* uses basal body temperature, cervical mucus, and cervical position to determine fertility. The most popular promoters of this method are the Couple to Couple League, which also publishes a magazine, *Family Foundations,* and offers peer support and professional consultation. (Disclosure: this author writes for *Family Foundations.*)

- *The Billings Ovulation Method* (Drs. John and Evelyn Billings) emphasizes the evaluation of cervical mucus patterns to determine fertility. The Billings Method is promoted by the Billings Ovulation Method Association — USA.

- *The Creighton Model* also relies on the evaluation of cervical mucus patterns, but is touted by Dr. Thomas Hilgers as an improvement upon the Billings Method (though the Billingses dispute this). The Creighton Model is promoted by the Pope Paul VI Institute at Creighton University in Omaha. The Pope Paul VI Institute also provides highly successful, morally licit, less expensive, and healthy alternatives to in vitro fertilization for couples who are struggling with infertility. They also offer a national network of physicians trained in this method known as Natural Procreative Technology (a.k.a. NaPro Technology).

- *The Marquette Method* employs an electronic fertility monitor (at this writing, the Clear Plan Fertility Monitor is the recommended device) to evaluate hormonal levels in the woman's urine stream (like a pregnancy test). Couples are taught to use this test, combined with other fertility signs, to recognize the signs leading up to ovulation. This method, which takes advantage of the most recent technology in fertility monitoring, is promoted by the Marquette University College of Nursing through its Institute for Natural Family Planning.

"Does everyone have to use NFP?"

Catholics are not required to use NFP. Instead, they may choose to use no method of family planning at all. This latter approach, called Providentialism, is a legitimate way for a couple to exercise their fertility.

That said, any couple who at some point in their relationship feels that it's necessary to space births or avoid pregnancy may use *only* one of the many forms of NFP available.

I would further argue that while the Church does not *require* couples to know NFP, that is a bit like saying that the Church does not require you to keep good financial records or eat right. No one is *required* by the Church to keep to a budget and maintain their checkbook, or maintain a healthy diet and exercise, but being a good steward of our financial resources — and bodies — is good and noble, and using those tools that empower us to do so is good and noble. In the same way, responsible parenthood *is* a requirement of the Church, and NFP is an outstanding tool for helping couples exercise good stewardship over their fertility. Moreover, even if a couple never feels the need or desire to use any means to postpone pregnancy, there may be times when knowledge of NFP actually helps a couple conceive. As millions of couples who struggle with primary and secondary infertility know, getting pregnant isn't always easy. So while it's true that couples are not obliged to use NFP, pastorally speaking, I believe most if not all couples may encounter a time in their marriage when they will feel handicapped without this tool in their toolbox.

"If contraception is so bad and NFP is so good, why is the Catholic Church the only Christian denomination that holds this position?"

The question would be more accurate if it were stated, "Why is the Catholic Church the only Christian denomination that *still* holds this position?" For 1,930 years, Christians — and many non-Christians — were unanimously against contraception. The following are some examples of people you might be surprised were opposed to contraception.

- *Martin Luther:* How great, therefore, the wickedness of human nature! How many girls there are who prevent conception and kill and expel tender fetuses, although procreation is the work of God! Indeed, some spouses who marry and live together ... have various ends in mind, but rarely children.

- *John Calvin:* The voluntary spilling of semen outside of intercourse between man and woman is a monstrous thing. Deliberately to withdraw from coitus that semen may fall on the ground is doubly monstrous. For this is to extinguish hope of the [human] race and to kill before he is born the hoped for offspring.

And, as you read earlier, this:

- *Mahatma Gandhi:* It is an insult to the fair sex to put up her case in support of birth-control by artificial methods. As it is, man has sufficiently degraded her for his lust and artificial methods ... will still further degrade her. I urge advocates of artificial methods to consider the consequences. ... Birth control to me is a dismal abyss.

Allan Carlson, writing in an issue of *Touchstone*, a magazine dedicated to dialog among the various Christian denominations (I have taken the quotations from Luther and Calvin from his articles), traces the *mainstream* Protestant opposition to contraception from the Reformers well into the twentieth century. Since the days of the Apostles, all of Christendom was united in its opposition to contraception, which was viewed as unbiblical and opposed to tradition until 1930, when the Anglicans voted at Lambeth to permit contraception, more as a concession to political and cultural pressures than anything else. After that, it was only a matter of time before all of Protestant Christianity, and even Orthodoxy, followed.

If the Catholic Church stands alone in affirming traditional Christianity and sanity in a world hell-bent on believing the crazy notion that the only way humanity can save itself is by preventing the next generation from being born, then I say it is the Catholic Church's honor and privilege to do so.

The good news, according to Carlson, is that after their eighty-year-long spiritual and mental leave of absence, Protestants are beginning to reclaim the historical Christian teaching on sexual morality. As R. Albert Mohler (who is, at this writing, president of the Southern Baptist Theological Seminary) told the *Chicago Tribune,* "It is clear that there is a major rethinking going on among Evangelicals on [contraception], especially among young people. There is a real push-back against the contraceptive culture now." Carlson also notes that the Family Research Council, an Evangelical Protestant family advocacy group, published a special report on "The Empty Promise of Contraception," and conservative Calvinist publishing houses are now promoting Natural Family Planning. As sociologist Andrew Greeley once wryly observed, Catholics have a knack for discarding Catholic practices just at the point when Protestants are beginning to discover their usefulness.

So rather than asking, "Why can't the Catholic Church get with all those other hip Christians who promote contraception?" it would be better, I think, to say, "I'm proud to be part of a tradition that kept that candle burning in the window so that others might eventually see the light."

"Contraception isn't forbidden in Scripture, is it?"

Contraception is forbidden in Scripture in Genesis 38:1–10, in which Onan, rather than fulfilling his obligation to provide his deceased brother with an heir, spills his seed on the ground, and is struck dead by God as punishment. Although some modern apologists from NACWATC try to deny the connection between this passage and contraception, these arguments are not rooted in the Christian tradition at all. For thousands of years, both Jewish and Christian scholars of all faiths viewed this passage as a direct condemnation of both masturbation and contraception.

According to *Catholic Sexual Ethics: A Summary, Explanation and Defense,* Catholics have also traditionally viewed scriptural prohibitions against patronizing witches and participating in witchcraft as condemnations of contraception and abortion. This is because, historically, witches claimed to have the power over life and death, and the main reason people went to visit the old village hag was not for the sometimes benign reasons for which superstitious and vulnerable people go to palm readers today, but rather to procure contraceptive potions, abortifacient potions, and other poisons. For instance, when St. Paul listed his denunciations of witchcraft *immediately after* his condemnations of specific sexual sins (see Gal. 5:19–21), early Christians understood exactly what he was talking about. Scriptural condemnations of witchcraft, according to Catholic scholarship, are in part condemnations of contraception and abortion.

Likewise, taken in light of God's positive command to be fruitful and multiply and the consistent view in Scripture that children are a blessing and a gift from God, the historical consensus among Christians has always been that, scripturally speaking at least, contraception is akin to spitting in God's eye.

"Are you saying I'm a bad person if I use contraception?"

Of course not. I have no doubt you're a good person trying to do the best you can with the life you have. I'm just saying you deserve better. You deserve to have options that enable you to take control of your fertility, not live in fear of it. You deserve to have better information than you've been given. Rather than having some pill shoved down your throat that risks your health (read the insert) and the health of your potential children (remember the Pill can cause miscarriage even after you're off it), you deserve to have *knowledge* that lets you discern when to have or not have a child in a manner that is healthy for you and your future child. The good news is there *are* other options that are much more respectful of your dignity as a person than contraception. Becoming aware of how you can use those options is an important part of taking responsibility for your life and your fertility as well as asserting that, as a son or daughter of God, your humanity is worth more than the makers of contraceptives would have you believe.

"Okay, so if contraception is so bad, why can't we just leave it to God?"

You can. As I wrote above, Providentialism is a legitimate option.

That said, while the desire to have a large family is admirable, it is difficult to imagine how one can know God's will in marriage or be totally open to it without regularly seeking that will in an ongoing prayerful relationship between a husband and wife. Some Christians (think of the Quiverful Movement) take the view that a couple doesn't need to pray about God's will for their family size because, having discerned the vocation to marriage, the couple is simply obliged to have as many children as possible.

I would argue that this attitude may well be contrary to Church teaching. As the *Catechism* tells us (CCC no. 2098): "Prayer is an indispensable condition for being able to obey God's commandments." Presumably this would also apply to God's command to be fruitful and multiply. Simply put, much as we might like one, there is no "one size fits all" approach to understanding or applying God's will. Every Christian couple, indeed, every Christian person, is called to live a holy life and actively seek God's will daily. A priest's prayerful discernment about the specifics of how he lives out his vocation (say, as a missionary, teacher, or pastor of a parish) cannot stop the day he is ordained, and neither can the prayerful discernment about how a married couple lives out their vocation stop the day they say "I do."

Furthermore, I would argue that there is a difference between "leaving it to nature" and "leaving it to God," a difference many people of good will fail to appreciate. Nature happens whether we pray about it or not, but God's will is revealed only by means of the prayerful and deliberate consideration of both grace and nature. In order to practice total openness to God's will, NFP-practicing couples prayerfully seek, each month, to understand both their bodily signs (nature) and how God is specifically calling them to live out their vocation *at this time* (grace). This is completely consistent with the Church's universal call to holiness and the teaching in *Gaudium et Spes,* no. 50, that it is the couple themselves who must decide "in the sight of God" whether to attempt to conceive or not in a given month. If that isn't a call to prayer, I don't know what is.

In short, the couple is free to practice Providentialism, but they are still obliged to practice it prayerfully and responsibly. To that end, NFP can help even those who are radically open to conception fulfill their calling.

"You seem to think that only couples who use NFP can be happy or virtuous. That isn't true!"

You're absolutely right. What's more, NFP is not a guarantee of happiness or virtue. But let's face it. People (and I speak for myself as much as anyone else) are lazy. Without some kind of accountability, people simply don't give as much priority to things such as sanctification, actualization, and intimacy. Even business consultant Stephen Covey argues as much in his popular self-improvement book *First Things First.* NFP provides the invitation and the accountability necessary to take the pursuit of virtue and intimacy in marriage seriously.

Beyond this, couples who use various forms of contraception are truly cheating themselves. Remember, when the Church says that contraception is a sin, she *means* that a couple is accepting so much less than God wants to give them. That's what sin is, ultimately — settling for less than the greatest good God wishes to give. Couples contracept for many reasons, including fear, marital problems, selfishness, laziness, ignorance, and immaturity, but none of those reasons promote intimacy or virtue. Remember, perfect (infallible) love casts out fear (1 John 4:18); it isn't facilitated by it. Saying that a contracepting couple is *capable* of being happy and virtuous is like saying people can smoke five packs a day and still be healthy. Maybe. But if they are, it will be in spite of a glaringly big, bad habit. Not because of it.

"Are you saying that NFP will 'divorce-proof' your marriage?"

Of course not. NFP is an invitation to participate in many good things, but it will benefit a couple only to the degree that they accept NFP's invitation to participate in all of those good things. If a couple practices the technical aspects of NFP, but ignores the invitation to prayer, communication, intimacy, and all the benefits promised by SPICE, choosing instead to ignore each other during the fertile time and white knuckle their way through until they can resume sex, then they will avoid the sin of contraception but little else. Rather than being Infallible Lovers, such a couple is engaging in sexual pharisaism in that they maintain the veneer of fidelity on the outside, but like "whitewashed tombs" are "full of death and dry bones" within (Matt. 23:27).

"I've heard a couple can only use NFP for 'grave reasons.'"

The phrase "grave reasons" comes from a popular — though flawed and unofficial — translation of *Humanae Vitae* that has caused much harm and misunderstanding. The official Vatican translation from the original Latin reads "serious reasons." What constitutes "serious reasons," however, is left to the couple to discern. Pope Pius XII indicated that the reasons a couple may choose to prevent pregnancy are "in truth, very wide." The Church asks only that every couple give prayerful consideration to "both their own welfare and that of their children, those already born and those which may be foreseen" as well as to exhibit a willingness to "reckon with both the material and the spiritual conditions of the times as well as their state of life ... [and] the interests of the family group, of temporal society, and of the Church herself" (*Gaudium et Spes*, no. 50).

"Nobody does NFP. Only 5 percent of Catholics use it!"

The pundits of the National Association of Conventional Wisdom on All Things Catholic (NACWATC) strike again! This argument is advanced as a way of suggesting that the Church's advocacy of NFP is a discredited teaching because "the sense of the faithful" opposes it. But the argument is hogwash.

First of all, if only 5 percent of people believed the earth was round, would that make it flat? Either something is true or it isn't. Polls don't change that. That said, let's take this question seriously and see where it leads us.

For the sake of argument, let's accept that Catholics who are observant of the Church's teaching on sexual morality in marriage constitute only 5 percent of the 66 million Catholics in America. What most people don't realize is that even if this is the case, then according to the *2004 National Council of Churches Yearbook,* there would be more sexually observant Catholics in America (3.3 million) than there are Episcopalians of any kind (2.3 million), Missouri-Synod Lutherans (2.5 million), Greek Orthodox (1.5 million), Church of Christ members (1.5 million), Jehovah's Witnesses (1 million), or Assemblies of God members (2.6 million). No one is suggesting that we should simply ignore what any of *these* groups have to say because of their small, and in many cases, shrinking numbers.

Taking this a bit further, accepting the 5 percent figure would mean that — if viewed, for purposes of comparison, as a separate denomination — Catholics who observed the Church's moral teaching on sexuality would constitute the tenth largest denomination in the United States, being just edged out for ninth place by Presbyterians (3.4 million).

No matter how you slice it, Catholics who observe Church teaching on sexual morality in marriage are not an insignificant group. In other words, "We're here. We're sincere. Get used to it."

"NFP is a new invention. What about all those generations that didn't have access to it? Adam and Eve didn't use NFP!"

This one is used by both progressives who like to poke a stick at what they think is the Church's NFP fetish and by ultra-conservatives who have a hard time separating NFP from contraception. Let's take this apart as quickly as possible.

Before the Fall, our first parents were in perfect harmony with God, each other, and nature. Their desires for each other and for children were perfectly ordered and responsible because they were united to God's love.

After the Fall, man suffered in many ways, and, sadly, many generations suffered greatly. For instance, many generations didn't have proper water treatment, or good nutrition, or antibiotics. So *nu?* The fact that past generations didn't have something is a lousy reason not to use it now.

"I know couples who say NFP damaged their relationship.
What do you have to say about that?"

The experience of these couples needs to be respected. In my position as a Catholic counselor who works with an almost exclusively Catholic population, the majority of whom are completely observant in matters of Catholic sexual teaching, I have encountered many couples who felt this way. But in my successful work with these couples, I've found that despite initial appearances, their issues rarely have anything to do with NFP and a great deal to do with the attitudes they bring to marriage about sex, communication, respect, spirituality, and self-control. Because this is an issue that warrants a thoughtful and serious response, I've dedicated an entire chapter to this problem in the section on overcoming common problems (see chapter 15).

"All this fussing over fertility is crazy.
I'm just going to get snipped and tied."

Whoa, whoa, whoa! Tell you what: whether we're talking about vasectomy or tubal ligation, why don't you just put down the knife before somebody gets hurt and let's talk, okay?

Do you really think that cutting out or cutting up parts of your body is the best response to your fears? Because, face it, if you're considering such a radical option, you're afraid of something. I don't know if you fear losing your mate if you get pregnant again, or if you're afraid for your health, or if you're afraid of jeopardizing your livelihood, or if you're afraid of something else, but maybe, just maybe, don't you think it would be better to address and overcome the problems causing those fears than to maim yourself in response to them?

You do realize, I hope, that sterilization doesn't prevent pregnancy 100 percent of the time. What will you do with your fears if, after having tried to bar, lock, shutter, and mutilate the door, life finds a way in anyway? Will you kill that life? Reject it?

Besides, what kind of a message does that send to your lover? I'll tell you what it says. "My body is mine, and I'm refusing to give you all of me. I am taking charge of my fertility. I don't care if you want it or not. I don't trust you to manage it with me. I am taking it away from you, and you can never have it again. My body. My choice." But this attitude is not only a serious offense to marital intimacy; it directly contradicts Scripture, which tells us that while the husband's body belongs to the wife and the wife's body belongs to the husband (1 Cor. 7:4), first and foremost, both belong to God (1 Cor. 6:18–20).

Sterilization takes what is intended to be holy — sex — and turns it into a radically selfish act that deprives the lovers of the full power of their love. Deal with your fears, and discover the truth. There is a responsible, safe, effective way to manage your fertility that doesn't require maiming yourself and depriving your lover of your whole self.

CONCLUSION

In this chapter, we've looked at NFP and found it to be a safe, effective tool that can be used to achieve or avoid pregnancy and to invite a couple to celebrate the deeper mysteries of Holy Sex.

Allow me to conclude by encouraging you to learn more. Even if you think you hate NFP, if you've never taken a course then you are — by definition — ignorant. Ignorance is not something to be proud of. At the very least, go learn something about the thing you think you hate so much. You might be surprised at what you find. Here are a few places you could begin your search.

Couple to Couple League, *www.ccli.org*
(800) 745-8252

Pope Paul VI Institute, *www.PopePaulVI.com*
(402) 390-6600

Marquette College of Nursing, *www.marquette.edu/nursing/NFP*
(414) 288-3800

Billings Ovulation Method Association – USA, *www.boma-usa.org*
(651) 699-8193

Books

The Art of Natural Family Planning: Student Guide, by Couple to Couple League International.

Merril Winstein. *Your Fertility Signals: Using Them to Achieve or Avoid Pregnancy Naturally.* St. Louis: Smooth Stone Press, 1989.

11 THE INFALLIBLE LOVER'S GUIDE TO PLEASURE

Hence it is that . . . words are set down that pertain to bodily love, so that the soul, wakened anew out of its listless state by a language to which it is accustomed, may heat up and may, by the language of a lesser love, be aroused to a higher. For in this book, kisses are mentioned, breasts are mentioned, cheeks are mentioned, loins are mentioned; and the holy pictures these words paint are not meant for mockery or laughter. Rather ought we focus our minds on the greater mercy of God. We must notice how marvelously and mercifully, in making mention of the parts of the body and thus summoning us to love, [God] works with us; for he reaches down into the vocabulary of our sensual love in order to set our hearts on fire, aiming to incite us to a holy loving. Indeed, by the act in which he lowers himself in words, he also elevates our understanding; for from the words associated with this sensual love we learn how fiercely we are to burn with love for the Divine.

—Pope St. Gregory the Great, On the Song of Songs

I have stated again and again that Holy Sex is highly pleasurable and beautifully sensual. As we discovered, Catholics offer Holy Sex as a positive option and antidote to the world's extremes. In the cultural marketplace, there are three entries competing for first place in the beauty pageant of sexual ideology. First, the Hedonists offer the Las Vegas Strip version of sex, with bright lights, flash, and noise serving as a paper-thin façade over the death, depression, estrangement, and isolation that dwells within.

In response to the Hedonists, the Negative Materialists offer their stripped down, duty-bound, airplane hangar view of sex. All function, no style, and certainly no sensuality, the Negative Materialists are suspicious not only of evil, but also of the glamour behind which evil often hides.

As a direct challenge to both of these extremes, Catholics submit their entry, Holy Sex as *Cathedral* — St. Peter's, Notre Dame, and the Basilica of the National Shrine of the Immaculate Conception all rolled into one, with all the smells and bells, sights and sounds, choirs and instruments, pomp and circumstance appropriate to a place where God's own love is made incarnate.

Infallible Lovers seeking to celebrate Holy Sex recognize the important role sensuality and erotic love play in celebrating the fullness of their passion together. In contrast to the Positive Materialists, though, who pursue pleasure and sensuality as an end in itself, leading to a hatred of the body, Infallible Lovers view eros as a means to an end, a tool facilitating the lovers' ability to be physical signs of God's love for each other and to cooperate with grace so that, as *Deus Caritas Est* states, they may transform and perfect each other in love.

Because of this, Infallible Lovers need never be suspicious of pleasure. For all the whining done in the popular media by members of NACWATC, you'd think there was a list of sexual prohibitions as long as the now defunct Index of Banned Books (ah, for the good old days...). Really, there is only One Rule Infallible Lovers need to be mindful of:

Every act of lovemaking must be respectful of the dignity of the couple and must express both an intention for greater unity and an openness to life.

Practically speaking, this means that a couple may do whatever they wish as long as both feel loved and respected and the marital act ends with the man climaxing inside the woman. That's it. That's the only rule, the One Rule. Everything else is left to the couple's prudential judgment.

SO YOU MEAN WE CAN DO WHATEVER WE WANT?

Although the Church is very generous when it comes to the pleasure a couple may enjoy in the pursuit of Infallible Loving, saying that something is left to the "prudential judgment" of the couple is not quite the same thing as saying "anything goes." Practically speaking, couples argue all the time about what they should or shouldn't do in the bedroom. Unfortunately, most of these arguments are never resolved because they are based on feelings rather than objective criteria that can guide a couple's discussions. Rather than prayerfully discerning how they may both respectfully and fully express their love for one another, too many couples cling to their own respective comfort zones and draw sexual boundaries based on preference as opposed to an honest commitment to be as loving, generous, and respectful as possible.

To that end, I would like to propose a few criteria couples may use to help guide their prudential judgment. After exploring those criteria together, I'll address some specific questions about sexual pleasure.

THE FOUR PLEASURE PRINCIPLES

Assuming that the One Rule is honored, I would encourage a couple struggling with disagreements about their sexual relationship to resist the temptation to root sexual discussions in their feelings — which may be influenced by many things that have nothing to do either with love or what's truly in the best interest of each other — and instead consider the following Four Pleasure Principles.

1. There should be continuity between your daily relationship and your sexual relationship.

2. While you should never be afraid to explore all the permitted pleasures, you should never be tempted to see each other merely as givers and receivers of pleasure. You must always respect the dignity of each other as persons.

3. Any sexual positions, items, articles of clothing, manners of speech, or playful actions used to help you achieve the fullness of sexual pleasure should be used in a manner that helps you and your beloved draw closer to each other, not to the thing. Things should never become the primary point of the sexual relationship. Rather, they

should be seen as the means you employ to experience the fullness of each other's love.

4. While a lover's comfort zones should not be the final arbiter in sexual disputes, feelings related to comfort zones must be respected. A lover's discomfort is reason enough to delay participating in some sensual activity, even if it is not enough to rule out entirely future participation in that activity. The couple should continue to evaluate all permitted pleasures in the light of the relationship and in a spirit of prayer.

Let's take a closer look at each of the Four Pleasure Principles used by Infallible Lovers in their celebration of Holy Sex.

1. *There should be continuity between your daily relationship and your sexual relationship.*

PHILIP AND ELIZABETH'S STORY

Philip and Elizabeth have been married for eighteen years, but they don't have a lot of time for each other. They both work long hours, and when they come home they try to make time for their kids. Weeks will go by before they have any conversations more significant than who has to pick up which kid or run what errand. Because they don't get a lot of time together, they are prone to misunderstanding each other's intentions and cues and tend to argue a fair amount. Some of those arguments are intense and, afterward, both feel resentful, but they rarely return to an argument to try to solve things after the fact. They just calm down, ignore the problem, and try to move on the best they can.

Generally, Philip and Elizabeth, although they are not at each other's throats, do not consider each other best friends. There are many things they don't feel comfortable discussing with each other. Philip doesn't discuss much with anyone, and Elizabeth has a few close women friends she shares things with.

Although theirs is not an intimate relationship, they spend a great deal of time focusing on their sex lives. Elizabeth and Philip usually have sex at least several times a week. Elizabeth has a large collection of sexy lingerie, and they have many different kinds of massage oils, sexual board games they play in the bedroom, and a few different vibrators that Philip uses on Elizabeth during foreplay or when he has climaxed before she has reached orgasm. They feel very close after sex and lean on it heavily to make up for the fact that they don't have a lot of time for each other during the day. According to both of them, their sex life is what keeps them going.

It may surprise you to know that, at least as their relationship is described above, it's not 100 percent clear that Philip and Elizabeth are technically doing anything that violates Catholic sexual teaching. As a counselor, I have grave pastoral concerns about this couple, however, because they are pretending to be a different, more intimate couple in the bedroom than they are in their everyday lives. This couple feels closer after sex, not because of increased emotional or spiritual intimacy, but because of the rush of hormones and neuro-transmitters that occurs after climax, which God has given us to *aid* intimacy, not stand in replacement of intimacy.

Scientists who study the process of human attachment tell us that sensory (i.e., physiological) attachment is important, but it is the weakest form of attachment. Attachment that is focused on emotional intimacy, mutual service, and cultivating a sense of belonging to each other is much deeper and more secure. The couple who focuses solely on sex to foster a sensory attachment to each other is attached, but tenuously so.

Technically, as far as Catholic moral teaching goes, there is nothing strictly forbidden about this approach to marriage, but that's only because the Church forbids all *sinful* actions, not all *stupid* ones. As we discussed in the chapter on eroticism, Holy Sex is driven by intimacy and assisted by arousal, whereas eroticism is simply about arousal. This couple is relying entirely too heavily on arousal and sensuality to keep their marriage together. Instead of their sexual relationship being a celebration of all that is good about their overall life together, their sexual relationship is at high risk for becoming the crutch on which their entire relationship leans.

The same goes for couples whose fantasy life involves pretending to be other people. Again, there's nothing wrong with injecting playfulness and even fantasy into the sexual relationship, assuming that those fantasies do not offend either the dignity of the lovers or objective moral principles. But what does it say about the couple's social intercourse — i.e., the close-ness they share all day long — if they're so bored with each other's daily relationship that they have to pretend to be strangers in the bedroom in order to feel aroused by each other?

The problem with Elizabeth and Philip is not that they enjoy sex. That is good. The problem is that they are using their sexual relationship as a drug that gets them through the day, using it to help them make up for the lack of time and energy they give to each other's hearts and souls all day long. If they continue this attitude, they run two risks over time. Either they will need to continue to pursue more and more dramatic/erotic experiences to make up for their lack of intimacy and their eventual accommodation to lesser sexual stimuli, or their sexual relationship will stagnate once they hit an erotic wall that one of them chooses not to cross or (according to the One Rule) shouldn't cross. In the latter event, individual spouses often get angry because the Church is mucking around in the bedroom. But the problem isn't the Church. The problem is the couple's unwillingness to accept the Church's invitation to strengthen their psychological and spiritual intimacy so that their *intimacy* will drive their sexual relationship, and so that there will be a continuity between their role of lovers in their daily relationship and their role as lovers in the bedroom.

> 2. *While you should never be afraid to explore all the permitted pleasures, you should never be tempted to see each other merely as givers and receivers of pleasure. You must always respect the dignity of each other as persons.*

Your spouse is a human being. Although your mate is capable of offering you much comfort and pleasure, your mate is not — nor is he or she ever intended to be — your sex toy. Any time you're tempted to think of each other merely as givers or receivers of pleasure, you're diminishing the personhood of your mate and the dignity of your marital relationship. As such, your sex life will suffer.

While your mate may be a source of great pleasure, you may never treat each other as vending machines where, if you push the right buttons, you have a right to be rewarded with whatever kind of sex you want, whenever you want it.

Imagine the following scenario. You've tried really hard to be loving to your mate all day. You've done some extra acts of service. You've tried to be more complimentary and casually affectionate throughout the day. Now the evening comes. Despite your best efforts to be attentive and loving, your mate is still very tired, and is not up to making love. Your mate proposes cuddling and falling asleep in your arms. How do you respond to this?

If you have a tendency to pout, withdraw, throw a tantrum, or become irritable and argumentative in light of not having all of your loving attention immediately rewarded, then despite any intentions you may have to the contrary, the simple fact is, you *are* treating your spouse as a vending machine. You pushed all the right buttons. Now, you deserve sex, and if you don't get it, you're going to complain to the manager.

Another example of viewing your spouse as merely a giver of pleasure and not a person is when you try to steamroll over your mate's objections when you would like to try certain positions or intimate acts in the bedroom but your spouse is not interested. We'll deal with this more under the Fourth Pleasure Principle, but for now, let's just say that it is inappropriate and unhelpful to respond to this refusal by trying to emotionally bully your mate (either through tantrums or pouting) to give you what you want.

In both cases, you're forgetting that your mate is a real person whom you have a positive obligation to love — that is, work for his or her good — whether you're getting paid for that love or not. Of course, you could attempt to have a respectful discussion that acknowledged your mate's exhaustion but then asked to plan the next opportunity to be intimate with each other before turning in for the night. But you don't have the right to ignore the personhood of your spouse in favor of your desire for pleasure *from* your spouse. This is what Pope John Paul II meant when he said that even married couples could commit adultery with each other. He took a lot of heat for that one from NACWATC, but he was right. Adultery is, essentially, the forsaking of real relationship so that people may use each other to provide whatever pleasure they can to one another. Obviously, this is not so far from how many married couples approach each other, and it's a problem on both a psychological and spiritual level.

So, by all means, enjoy your mate and all the pleasure you can find in your spouse's arms. Just remember that your mate is not a vending machine to kick if you don't always get what you want. Rather, your mate is a person who deserves your love and service even when sex isn't offered as payment for services rendered.

> 3. *Any sexual positions, items, articles of clothing, manners of speech, or playful actions used to help you achieve the fullness of sexual pleasure should be used in a manner that helps you and your beloved draw closer to each other, not to the thing. Things should never become the primary point of the sexual relationship. Rather, they should be seen as the means you employ to experience the fullness of each other's love.*

Having a playful sexual relationship is a wonderful thing, but the point of Holy Sex is celebrating intimacy, not planning an event. In the course of celebrating their intimacy, Infallible Lovers should by all means feel free to use whatever sexual positions, lingerie, passionate speech, and other resources might help them draw closer to each other and experience the fullness of the passion they have for one another. Sometimes, however, a couple can get to the place where unless X *thing* happens, the sex "doesn't count."

FRANK AND BRENDA'S STORY

"I love it when we go down on each other during foreplay," says Frank, expressing how much he enjoys it when he and his wife, Brenda, orally stimulate

each other leading up to intercourse. "There's just something so intimate and beautiful about being free to kiss every part of each other's bodies. I love the way she looks when she opens herself up to me. I love the way she tastes, and I love seeing her kiss and stroke me too. It feels so good and it means so much to me. Like she's really just crazy in love with all of me and vice versa.

"The problem is, sometimes she just isn't into it, and she just wants to cuddle and then move right to intercourse. That's okay, I guess. But it's just not the same. I just feel like I'm being cheated if we don't do that. I feel like she's holding out, and I really don't enjoy sex nearly as much."

Frank's feelings are easy to understand; we all know a man or woman who says something similar. But Frank is violating the third pleasure principle, and very likely the second one as well. As long as Frank and Brenda observe the *One Rule*, requiring the man to climax inside the woman, there's nothing wrong with Frank's enjoyment of oral stimulation during foreplay. Many people enjoy the intensity of the sensations and the intimacy conveyed by it. The problem is when Frank feels cheated if that action isn't part of the particular sexual experience. It was not surprising that his wife said to me in a subsequent session, "I actually like doing that [giving and receiving oral stimulation] with him, but I feel like I'm going to be punished if I don't. He gets all upset and he whines about it. He makes me feel like my performance wasn't good enough. I don't want to *perform* for him. I want to *love* him, and I don't want to be punished for not following his damn script every single time. I'm a real person, not some woman he hired to jump through his hoops. And I resent being treated like one."

Brenda is right to be upset. Frank has turned what could have been a loving and intimate part of their sexual relationship into the entire point of their sexual relationship. As a result, Brenda feels objectified and demeaned by an action that, in and of itself, is not necessarily objectifying or demeaning. It is Frank's attitude toward this activity that is offensive, not the activity itself.

Any time a husband or wife allows one part of their lovemaking to become the entire point of their lovemaking, they obliterate the intimacy of intercourse and turn each other into mere givers or receivers of pleasure instead of persons deserving of love. As a result, defensiveness increases and boundaries go up as the partners try to protect themselves from being used by each other.

In your relationship, you should feel free to enjoy all the permitted pleasures that allow you to express your love for each other fully, but you must be careful to avoid falling more in love with a particular pleasure than with each other. Otherwise, there's a great risk that your mate will feel like you are refusing to make love because you're too interested in having an affair with a technique.

4. *While a lover's comfort zones should not be the final arbiter in sexual disputes, feelings related to comfort zones must be respected. A lover's discomfort is reason enough to delay participating in some sensual activity, even if it is not enough to rule out entirely future participation in that activity. The couple should continue to evaluate all permitted pleasures in the light of the relationship and in a spirit of prayer.*

In lesser marriages, spouses decide how loving to be toward one another based upon their comfort zones. This is a dynamic that holds true for every aspect of the relationship, not just the sexual relationship. When a wife in such a relationship asks a husband to go to church with her, be more communicative or more expressive, or any other thing that may ask more of him than he cares to give, the husband rejects the invitation with the excuse "that just isn't me." When a husband in such a relationship asks the wife to be more physically affectionate, watch the big game with him, or help him with some project, the wife will reject the invitation with a similar excuse. In either case, these husbands and wives tend to place a higher value on protecting their own comfort zones than in pursuing deeper intimacy.

In *For Better . . . FOREVER!* I argue that such an attitude may be acceptable for secular marriage, but it flies in the face of the ideals guiding

Christian marriage. Christian marriage is founded upon the principle that the husband and wife have an important role to play in God's plan for perfecting each other in love. God gives you the particular husband or wife he has given you so that you'll be challenged to grow in ways that neither of you would ever think of if you were left to your own devices. When your partner expresses the desires of his or her heart — assuming that the request does not violate objective moral principles or your dignity as a person — I encourage you to view that as an opportunity to respond positively to the invitation God has written to you on your mate's heart, so that you may grow in ways that will enable you to become the person God created you to be. In the course of a marriage, God may call you, through the needs and desires he has written on your mate's heart, to grow in many ways that, at first, make you uncomfortable. But if you respond to God's invitation, expressed to you through your mate's request, you'll become a better person, a more competent lover, and a more effective servant of God. But if, instead, you choose to cling to your own comfort, you will simply not grow, and your marriage may stagnate. You'll be like the servant who buries his treasure — your very self — in the ground rather than risking anything.

That said, as one spouse struggles to respond to the other spouse's request, the other is obliged to be patient, understanding, supportive, and sympathetic. This is the receiving spouse's opportunity to grow in generosity and patience as he (or she) resists the temptation to tap his toe, keep glancing at the time, and periodically exclaim, "You're *still* struggling with this? Yeesh!" The receiving spouse is obliged to find ways to reach out to the mate who is struggling to be more giving. It is the receiving spouse's job to be compassionate and say, "Thank you for extending yourself and working so hard to love me. What can I do to lighten your load or help you through whatever difficulties you're having with taking on this new role?"

If this is true of Infallible Lovers in their day-to-day relationship, it's doubly true of Infallible Lovers in their sexual relationship. When your spouse asks you to expand your sexual repertoire beyond your immediate comfort zone, I encourage you to understand your spouse's desire as God's invitation to you to grow in new ways to express God's own complete, total, unreserved passion for your mate. It's an opportunity for you to grow to new levels of generosity and intimacy. You can choose to hide behind your sexual comfort zone, in which case your physical relationship will be strained as the result of your decision to cling to your preferences over the call to love as an Infallible Lover. If, on the other hand, you choose to respond to the invitation, you'll grow into a more intimate lover and a better physical sign of God's own love for your mate. This is why evaluating any new permissible sexual ideas that challenge a mate's comfort zones should be done prayerfully. Infallible Lovers are not merely loving each other; they are representing God's love to and for each other.

Nonetheless, like with the struggle to become more loving in every other aspect of your relationship, you do need to be respectful to each other's sexual comfort zones. Asking a mate to challenge his or her comfort zone for the sake of love is different from demanding that they deliver on some request immediately. Infallible Lovers don't use their own comfort zones as the final arbiter of disputes about whether or not to grant a particular request; they defer instead to the virtues that they are called to exhibit in their marriage and objective moral principles. Still, they do work hard to be patient with each other when growth is difficult or takes longer than either spouse would prefer.

It is enough that your mate is willing to work to develop competency and greater comfort with whatever it is you're asking them to do. Your role will be to find ways to be supportive, to ask how you might help your mate feel more confident about the steps being taken, to be more encouraging and loving in every area of your relationship so that your mate can be safe taking this risk, and sometimes, to let your spouse off the hook for not fulfilling a request that's just too difficult on a given day. By being supportive and patient and even by generously sacrificing your desires on those days when your mate just isn't up to the challenge, you make it that much easier for your mate to try harder to be everything you need and want him or her to be — everything God himself needs you to be to each other.

PUTTING IT ALL TOGETHER: A CASE STUDY

It might seem difficult to apply these four principles in practice, so let's look at a case study. Cherrie and Adam attended one of my talks on Holy Sex and spoke with me afterward about some concerns they'd been having. Overall, their relationship seemed solid, but they were having a sexual issue that they wanted some counseling for. We conducted six sessions over the phone over the course of three months.

Cherrie and Adam have been married for four years. They have two children and they love each other very much. They work hard to take time each day to talk with each other about how well they are attending to each other's spiritual and emotional needs, and they take regular prayer time as a couple as well as with their children. They also work hard to find little ways to reach out to each other throughout the day. They call each other from work to keep each other apprised of their schedules and goings-on, and they are not shy about saying "I love you" and being physically affectionate. They often write short notes to each other, or bring each other flowers or other little tokens of their affection for one another.

Generally speaking, their sexual relationship is satisfying. Adam and Cherrie try hard to remember that their sexual relationship is not just a celebration of their love and partnership, but a way that God makes his own love for each of them incarnate.

It surprised Adam, then, one night when they were making love, when he asked Cherrie to try a new sexual position — one that would involve her kneeling and facing away from him while he entered her from behind — that she became angry and refused. He was hurt and frustrated. He hadn't meant to offend her, but she was adamant. They ended up breaking off their lovemaking and going to bed angry and confused.

The next evening, during the time they regularly took to pray together and discuss how well they had been attending to each other spiritually and emotionally that day, they tried to talk through their reactions to each other the night before.

202

Cherrie explained that she felt degraded. That she liked being able to look into Adam's eyes when they made love, and that this just made sex feel anonymous. Also, although Cherrie didn't consider herself to hold many feminist pretensions, the position just seemed too submissive, and the fact that some people refer to it as "doggy style" just made it seem animalistic and wrong.

For his part, Adam said that he wasn't thinking of any of those things when he asked her to try the new position. He said that he understood where she was coming from, but that he saw it differently. He said that when he thought of making love to her that way, he imagined seeing her opening up to him completely; being able to watch her draw him into her and being able to hold her breasts, and even whisper into her ear and kiss her neck and back, seemed to him very intimate and passionate. He said he understood her point about the position being submissive, and he said that he understood why she would be intimidated by that if she regularly felt that he was trying to take advantage of her or control or manipulate her in their daily relationship. But if she didn't feel that way, then maybe the submission represented by that position could just be an extension of her letting him love and serve her all day long.

Cherrie said she hadn't thought about it that way before, but she still felt somehow "wrong" about trying it. Adam said that he could respect that, but he reminded her that there wasn't anything objectively immoral about the new position, and he asked her to at least think about it, and try not to judge him for still wanting her to try it.

Over the course of the next few weeks, they made love several times without trying the new position. Adam didn't pressure Cherrie, but they kept discussing her concerns about it during their nightly couple time. After having the chance to reflect on it, and even pray about it together, Cherrie conceded that she realized there were lots of small ways that she fought Adam when he tried to take care of her, because she didn't want to be "too dependent or submissive." For instance, sometimes if Cherrie was busy with the kids and Adam would offer to do the household tasks she considered "her jobs," she would become angry and defensive. She felt like he was taking over, like he was saying she couldn't handle things, but she realized this was irrational. Adam had demonstrated time and again that he loved her and had no desire to control her. He just wanted to help. She realized that she was holding on to old fears that she learned from her mom and dad. Dad was kind of controlling, and after her mom and dad split up, Cherrie had promised herself she would never become too dependent on "some man." She didn't think about it much these days, but on some level, she recognized that she was letting this childish oath put distance between her and Adam in a lot of different areas of her relationship.

It occurred to her that her anger over Adam's suggestion to try the new position was representative of her larger concerns about just letting go and being loved by Adam. They agreed to try to work together on her being more open to his efforts to practice servant-leadership first in their daily life together, and then they'd see what happened in the bedroom. Adam would continue to look for ways to step in and help when she was overwhelmed by other responsibilities, and in return she would work hard to let him take care of her and submit to his loving service.

After trying this over the course of a few weeks, Cherrie found that she was not only becoming more comfortable with Adam's offers of help, she was also surprised to find herself almost spontaneously warming up to the idea of the new position. One morning, when she was just waking up but still half asleep, she found herself fantasizing about him taking her the way Adam had described weeks before. Only this time, instead of feeling threatened and demeaned by it, she felt swept up, taken care of. She loved the idea of allowing him to take control of her body and love her, just as he was willing to, in a sense, "stand behind her" when she needed his care throughout the day. That morning, she whispered to Adam that she had a surprise for him that night, but she wouldn't tell him what. Later that evening, after the kids were asleep, she put on some lingerie and began cuddling with Adam. When it was time to make love, Adam started to get into their usual position, but Cherrie stop him and asked him to wait. Adam was confused at first, and a little worried, but his fears evaporated quickly as he watched Cherrie get into the position she and Adam had been discussing weeks before. Feeling nervous and vulnerable and excited all at once, she told Adam to make love to her like he had described he would that first night.

They both agreed that that night was truly special. Cherrie and Adam continue to make love both in the more familiar ways as well as trying new things.

But by taking the time to explore Cherrie's fears, consider their sex life in the context of their whole relationship, and (while respecting each other's feelings) refusing to allow feelings to dictate the sexual relationship, Cherrie and Adam discovered new ways to be intimate to each other in and out of the bedroom.

WHAT CHERRIE AND ADAM CAN TEACH US

Cherrie and Adam's story highlights several important points. First of all, this couple worked hard to apply the first pleasure principle: continuity. They refused to simply treat their sexual relationship as separate from their daily relationship. Realizing that the way they related sexually said something about the way they related to each other in their day-to-day life, they knew that any concerns about their sex life had to be rooted in their wider interactions. They did a good job of pinning down those problems, and instead of nagging each other they trusted that by working to improve certain aspects of their daily relationship — specifically their cooperation and partnership — their sexual relationship would also improve.

Second, Cherrie and Adam did an excellent job of remembering the second pleasure principle: resist the temptation to reduce each other to merely givers and receivers of pleasure. Although Adam could have pouted and become angry himself for Cherrie's defensive attitude and re-fusal to accommodate his request, he did a good job of remembering that Cherrie was a person who deserved to be heard and understood. For her part, after she had had time to reflect more deeply on her feelings and beliefs, Cherrie did a good job remembering that Adam was not some per-vert, but a good man who deserved — by nature of his love and service to her — a fair hearing and the benefit of the doubt. Rather than simply treating the exchange as a failed attempt to give and receive pleasure, they mined the experience for the meaning and intimacy that was buried within.

Next, Cherrie and Adam used the third pleasure principle. Although Adam did want to be able to try the new position with Cherrie, he didn't make their entire sexual relationship about trying that new position. He didn't make her feel like a failure for her hesitancy. He recognized that being intimate was the most important thing, more important than having new experiences. While he wanted Cherrie to be more open to new experiences, he knew that the only way to help her through her concerns was to build on the foundation of all the good they already had going in their relationship, not browbeating her and making her feel incomplete because she refused to follow his script.

Finally, Adam and Cherrie did well employing the fourth pleasure principle. They respected Cherrie's feelings while not letting either person's comfort zone be the final arbiter of whether it would be appropriate to try the new position. Instead, they allowed objective moral principles and the larger context of their marital relationship help them determine whether the increased vulnerability represented by this new position was safe or not.

PROBLEM-SOLVING
WITH THE FOUR PLEASURE PRINCIPLES

The same process can be used to resolve almost any sexual difference of opinion between married couples — whether about different positions, activities during foreplay, frequency of intercourse, or other issues. In this sense, the four pleasure principles are actually a frontline problem-solving format. It outlines a process by which couples can safely explore all the possible ways they can increase their intimacy and enjoyment of each other in and out of the bedroom.

When you are negotiating some aspect of your sexual relationship (whether issues related to frequency or suggestions regarding new techniques or other additions to your sexual repertoire), consider the following steps that have been outlined in this chapter.

1. Ask yourselves: does this new suggestion or idea violate the One Rule? (If so, then the discussion is essentially over because it is either objectively immoral or personally demeaning.)

2. Assuming it does not violate the One Rule, pray about the new idea. Does the proposed improvement or addition to your sexual relationship make sense in the larger context of the way you and your mate relate to each other? That is, does the respect, intimacy, attention, affirmation, affection, and partnership you display all day make it safe and appropriate to try to incorporate this new idea into your sexual relationship?

   • If "yes," then move on to step 3.

   • If "no," then ask, "What steps can we take to improve the respect, intimacy, attention, affirmation, affection, and partnership we share throughout the day so that incorporating this new idea into our sexual relationship makes more sense?" Address this, then move to step 3.

3. "How will we make sure that this new idea doesn't become the entire focus of our lovemaking instead of simply being one of the many means we have at our disposal to enjoy greater intimacy?"

4. If one of you is uncomfortable introducing the new suggestion into your sexual relationship, consider the following:

   • Is the discomfort you're experiencing the result of feeling that the vulnerability caused by incorporating this new suggestion is somehow inappropriate given the level of respect, intimacy, attention, affirmation, affection, and partnership you currently share in your relationship overall? If "yes," return to step 2 and answer the questions there.

     OR

   • Is the discomfort you're experiencing the result of old personal baggage that has little or nothing to do with your present relationship?

- If "yes," then discuss: "What steps will I take to work through these personal obstacles to intimacy, and what support will I need from my spouse while I work through these issues?"

- Also, revisit the questions under step 3.

The steps outlined in this chapter offer objective criteria that can help you successfully negotiate sexual disagreements that would otherwise get bogged down in subjective discussions about comfort zones and personal preferences. By following these steps, you can make sure that you're being both as generous and as moral and respectful as possible as you pursue the fullness of sexual intimacy and pleasure in your marital relationship.

12

THE ANATOMY OF
INFALLIBLE LOVING:
SETTING THE STAGE

*I know that my words embarrass many of you, and the reason for your
shame is your own wanton licentiousness. . . . Why else would you be
ashamed at what is honorable or blush at what is undefiled? That is
why . . . I want to restore marriage to its proper nobility and to silence
those heretics who call it evil. . . . Some of you call my words immodest
because I speak of [sex] which is honorable; . . . but by calling my words
immodest you condemn God, who is the author of marriage.*

—St. John Chrysostom, from his homilies on sex and marriage

This chapter and the following chapter build upon everything we
have discussed up to this point. There are essentially four stages of
Holy Sex.

1. Social Intercourse
2. Foreplay
3. Sexual Intercourse
4. Afterglow

This chapter will provide information on the basics of social intercourse
and foreplay. The next chapter will examine how to get the most out of
intercourse itself as well as the all-important but much neglected afterglow.
Together these two chapters will serve as an extended exercise that you
and your mate can use to get to know yourselves and each other a little
better. By the conclusion of this chapter and the next, you will have
what you need to master the art of being exceptional Infallible Lovers,
celebrating an eros that empowers you to rise up to touch the Divine.

SOCIAL INTERCOURSE

Social intercourse refers to the intimacy you share throughout the day in your relationship. As we've noted, Infallible Lovers do not ignore each other all day long, only to roll over, face each other in bed, and out of the blue ask "So, you wanna do it?" Infallible Lovers recognize that everything they do together must be infused with passion, intimacy, and partnership. In this way, the Infallible Lovers' sexual relationship becomes a celebration of everything that is already good in their marriage, not merely the sensual glue that holds a tenuous bond together.

Although my previous book *For Better...FOREVER!* touches on matters of sexuality, it is primarily concerned with increasing a couple's capacity for social intercourse. Readers who would like to delve deeper into problem-solving, effective communication, and marital spirituality would do well to go there for a more thorough look at this topic.

That said, this book would not be complete without offering some suggestions for improving the most important part of a couple's sexual relationship. If a couple does not share deep intimacy, close communication, and abundant affection and affirmation in their day-to-day relationship, then instead of representing the fruit of their loving, their sexual relationship will seem like something awkwardly grafted on to the tree of their lives together.

We broadly addressed the topic of social intercourse in our discussion on NFP and sexual intimacy. In that section, you were introduced to the acronym SPICE, which refers to the couple's care for the Spiritual, Physical, Intellectual, Creative, and Emotional dimensions of their relationship (see above, p. 172). The following represent some of the most important tips for attending to these aspects of your marriage.

Rituals and Routines

A study published in the journal *Family Process* examined fifty years of research on the importance of rituals and routines for the health of marriage and family life. Researchers found that couples and families who have committed regular time to daily and weekly activities such as prayer time, family meal times, family game nights, regular time for couples to talk and share, worship time, family days, couple's dates, etc., are significantly stronger and happier and are at significantly lower risk for divorce, depression, and mental illness, behavioral and school problems in children, and a host of other problems, when compared to couples without such rituals. In fact, research shows that rituals and routines are almost more important than the actual composition of a family. On average, families who suffer the loss of a member to death or divorce, but maintain their weekly rituals and routines, are healthier and more satisfied with their relationships than intact couples and families without these routines.

Furthermore, couples who commit themselves to maintaining the routines even during conflict have much more stable relationships than those who don't. If a couple is angry with each other, but have committed to their meal times, prayer times, playful times, and communication times, even though these times might not be as fruitful as when they are getting along, they are communicating an important message to each other: "You can count on me to be here for you even when things get tough."

Couples who refuse to participate in their routines when they are in conflict send a different message. They are saying, "Conflict can throw our whole relationship into question. Unless everything is perfect, don't count on me to be here for you."

It should be obvious that these different messages have a profound effect on each couple's sexual relationship.

Take a moment to reflect on the following areas of your life together. What steps could you take to improve the rituals and routines that bind you together?

Spirituality

- Write down some examples of how you would like to grow closer together spiritually. Examples include actions like weekly or daily Mass, daily prayer time as a couple and family, Scripture and spiritual reading, and learning more about devotions you can share. (A great resource for other ideas is the *How To Book of Catholic Devotions* by Regis Flaherty and Mike Aquilina.)

- Now list changes that you and your spouse would need to make to increase the likelihood of following through on these activities.

Connection

Another area facilitated by rituals and routines is the connection between a couple. Holy Sex is a celebration of the intimacy and connection a couple already enjoys throughout the day. Rituals that improve couple connection include family meal time, daily talking time, calling each other throughout the day just to say, "I love you," planning your schedules with your marriage and family in mind, working on projects together, and being better partners to each other. (Do not include fun activities here. We will deal with those next.)

- What daily or weekly activities might help you feel more connected to your spouse?

- What changes would you and your spouse need to make to increase the likelihood of following through on these activities?

Playfulness

Holy Sex is playful and pleasurable, but a couple can't be all business all day long and then suddenly expect to have a playful, joyful sexual relationship when they get into bed together. In order for a couple's sexual relationship to be as joyful as it can be, the couple must have regular times when they're playful with each other throughout the day. Examples of playful rituals include game nights, sharing hobbies, looking for ways to inject humor into the jobs you do together, family day, and date nights.

- Write down your ideas for rituals that would help you and your mate increase the playfulness in your day-to-day relationship.

- What changes would you and your spouse need to make to increase the likelihood of following through on these activities?

Your commitment to the activities you listed in the categories above will help you maintain closeness and continuity between your daily life and your sexual relationship.

The Daily Marital Checkup

The Daily Marital Checkup is another way to improve your social intercourse. This is a simple exercise that helps you both evaluate how well you are attending to each other and your marriage from day to day. It also gives you a positive way to ask one another for help attending to various spiritual, emotional, and psychological needs.

The Daily Marital Checkup consists of these two questions:

1. What did we do to try to attend to each other's spiritual and emotional needs today?

2. What can we do to attend to each other even better tomorrow?

These questions challenge couples to go deeper than the usual conversations about who is going to run what errand and what child needs to be picked up when. If you aren't used to thinking on this level, here are examples of ways you can attend to each other's spiritual and emotional needs:

- Taking time to pray for each other before the big meeting or difficult confrontation with a friend.

- Making sure to make a little extra time for each other when one of you is feeling stressed.

- Doing those extra, unexpected small acts of service, just because you wanted to lighten your mate's load today (see the Lovelist exercise just below).

- Bringing home some token of affection, just because you wanted to make your mate's life a little easier or more pleasant.

- Making sure to call each other several times a day while at work or on a business trip, just to stay connected and manage each other's expectations about your moods and your plans for when you get together again.

- Remembering to ask about those things you know are weighing heavily on your mate's heart — whether you are particularly concerned about those things or not — and trying to do things to alleviate these concerns without being asked.

Exercise
THE LOVELIST

One of the simplest yet most powerful exercises I describe in *For Better . . . FOREVER!* and use with my clients is the Lovelist exercise. The exercise consists of writing down at least twenty-five nonsexual things that make you feel loved when your mate does them for you. The Lovelist is not a complaint list. Couples are not allowed to write down things they wish their mate would stop doing or that they would like to change about their mate's personality. The Lovelist is simply a list of those thoughtful things that your mate has done, does do, or you wish they would do more of that make you feel loved on a gut level. I write, "make you feel loved on a gut level" because the things you write should give that gut-feeling that says, "Gosh! That was really nice! You didn't have to do that! Thank you!" The items you list should not take a lot of time, or cost a lot of money. They are just thoughtful, simple acts of service or affection that are personally meaningful to you.

Examples of what you might include on your Lovelist include, "I feel loved when I come home and the garbage is already at the curb," or, "I feel loved when you call me to tell me you love me," or, "I feel loved when you get my favorite ice cream even though you don't like it," or, "I feel loved when you hug me — just because."

Come up with your own Lovelist by completing this sentence:

I feel loved throughout the day when you. . . .

Once you have your Lovelists, trade them with your mate. Each day, challenge yourselves to do something on your mate's Lovelist. Try your best to do at least one thing that is easy for you to do, and one thing that is a bit of a stretch for you. Discuss your efforts in your Daily Marital Checkup.

Next let's look at your transition from social intercourse into your sexual relationship.

FOREPLAY

Despite what secular sex therapists might tell you, foreplay is about more than getting the blood pumping and the juices flowing. For Infallible Lovers, foreplay is the bridge on the road from daily intimacy to sexual intimacy. While social intercourse is not separate from sexual intercourse, even couples who are generally attentive to their social intercourse find that the degree of closeness in their daily relationship can wax and wane based on unexpected stressors, obligations, and the crises that are common to family life. The first purpose of foreplay is to serve as a kind of decompression chamber that allows you to check in with each other and make sure that the transition from partners to lovers will be a smooth one. The second purpose of foreplay is to set the stage for the sacred mystery that allows your love for one another to be incarnate. Let's take a look at these dimensions of foreplay.

The Bridge to Sexual Intimacy

As we noted above, foreplay serves as the bridge that transitions you from intimate partners to passionate lovers. In this sense, before you and your spouse begin to kiss or touch each other in any way, it is good to take a moment to make sure that your relational and spiritual connection is secure. Take a moment to pray together and do your Daily Marital Checkup (p. 213). New moms especially complain that they can find it difficult to make the transition from mother to vixen. Taking time to remind each other, first, of the ways you've been trying to take care of each other all day every day and, second, of the spiritual significance of your lovemaking, can be helpful in easing this transition.

Use your Marital Checkup to make sure you know where each of you is starting psychologically, spiritually, and relationally. If your mate has had a difficult day, you may need to be more sensitive and, perhaps, be more of the initiator, in any lovemaking. This may also be a time to stick to familiar and comfortable patterns of lovemaking. Or, if your spouse is in a wonderful place psychologically, spiritually, and relationally, this might be the time to try something new and be more playful and adventurous. Taking time to check in with each other emotionally and spiritually — however briefly — will help prevent those disagreements that can occur when one lover is expecting fireworks while the other is hoping for something quiet and tender. Plus, you will make certain that your lovemaking is rooted in authentic intimacy and an eros that enables you to rise up toward the Divine.

Setting the Stage for the Banquet

The second purpose of foreplay is to set the stage for the sacred mystery that allows your love for one another to become incarnate.

Recall that when we explored the First Power of Holy Sex: the power to make the common holy, we drew a direct connection between the Eucharist and the sacrament of matrimony. In both instances, love becomes incarnate. In the former instance, love becomes incarnate when, in the words of the Easter Vigil prayer, "Heaven is wedded to earth" and the bread and wine become the Real Presence, the Body and Blood of Jesus Christ. In the latter instance, love becomes incarnate when husband and wife express with their bodies the spiritual reality of the unity, partnership, and love they share but otherwise could not see. As Pope John Paul II observed in The Theology of the Body, it is the body that has been given the power by God to make visible that which is invisible.

Likewise, as you discovered in our examination of the First Power of Holy Sex, the Church is not shy in making a direct and powerful connection between the Eucharist, the ultimate marital act, and sexual intercourse, the "primordial sacrament."

"So," you might ask, "what does any of this have to do with foreplay?"

Everything.

The couple celebrating their incarnational sacrament (Holy Sex in marriage) should take their cue from how the Church celebrates *the* incarnational sacrament, the "summit and source of our faith," the Eucharist. "Say what!" you exclaim. I know, I know. Stop hyperventilating and think about this a minute.

The Church celebrates the sacred mysteries in beautifully adorned spaces, employing special clothing that adds to the drama and beauty of the moment, music that lifts the soul, and scents that remind us of heavenly love. The Mass is *supposed* to be a scandalous feast of the senses (ask any Puritan) specifically intended to remind us of that most scandalous reality — how Christ, by becoming one flesh with nature, makes all matter Divine. The Mass is the wedding supper of the Lamb. All of the smells, bells, music, attire, pomp, and ceremony are intended as a kind of spiritual foreplay that sets the stage for the consummation of the marriage between the bride (us) and the bridegroom (Jesus Christ) when we receive the precious Body and Blood and we become one flesh with God. There are those who will struggle with this kind of language and imagery, but I'm afraid there's no getting around it. This is the authentic Catholic vision of the Mass. And no matter how odd this vision may seem to you, husbands and wives can learn a lot from the Church about the process that is the dramatic build-up to intimate union.

Just as the Church is not shy about celebrating the sensual in its sacrament of incarnational divine love, the couple celebrating the sacred mysteries of their marital love should not be shy about engaging all the senses as they set the stage for their becoming one flesh with each other.

Foreplay helps you engage all of your senses and prepares your body to be intimately aware of the other so that you can give yourselves completely to each other and receive each other completely in return. Assuming that we are rooting lovemaking in its proper spirituality and relationality, the more sensual foreplay is, the more spiritual the entire experience of lovemaking can ultimately be: foreplay is your way of waking up all the senses so that each lover's body can receive the other wholly.

I don't mean to imply that every act of Holy Sex must be a festival of the senses. To continue our analogy, there are High Masses and Low Masses. There are great feast day Masses, and there are simple, quiet, daily Masses. All of them are celebrations of incarnational love, and each is beautiful and sensual in its own way. In the same way, Holy Sex can be earth-shattering, or it can be simple and quiet, but it will always be sensual. Infallible Lovers should not be afraid to be as fully sensual as they can, and as is permitted, in preparing to celebrate the sacred mysteries of their love for one another.

With that in mind, I would like to ask you to consider how you can more fully employ your sacred senses of taste, smell, sight, hearing, and touch in preparing each other to celebrate that sacrament of incarnational love known as Holy Sex. As you consider being more sensual in your foreplay — and subsequently lovemaking — remember that the point of sensuality is *not* simply to be sensual. The point is to heighten the senses so that each of you is empowered to give yourself more fully and receive each other more completely in return. Let's examine ways that you can increase your experience of each other through your senses during foreplay — both to increase the pleasure of the experience and to discover more ways to reveal yourselves to one another.

Taste and Smell

Let us ... offer a honeycomb at the table of the Lord in the heavenly [wedding] banquet. . . . How splendid also is the fragrance of faith in all these mysteries! (St. Bernard of Clairvaux, On the Song of Songs)

While our senses of taste and smell may not be as central in advanced stages of foreplay and intercourse, they are important to setting the stage and preparing to make an attractive gift of ourselves to our lover.

Our senses of taste and smell remind us that the simple things matter when entering into the sacred mysteries of incarnational love. Taking time to make sure your breath is sweet and that your body is clean and fresh are important ways of showing respect for yourself, your lover, and the sacredness of Holy Sex. As we learn from the Bible, purifying rituals are always tied to sacred acts. Wash up, spruce up, and take a moment to purify yourself for the sacred act of love.

Likewise, just as the Church uses incense at Mass to put us in mind of the sweet scent of heaven coming down to earth, simple things like a touch of cologne or perfume and a lightly scented candle can take you out of the banality of your daily circumstances and make an ordinary space seem extraordinary. The book of Esther (2:12) discusses the preparations of myrrh, perfumes, and cosmetics that would be used to prepare a queen for her wedding day with the king. We who are sons and daughters of God should take care to prepare our bodies so that they will be fresh and sweet-smelling and we can present ourselves to our lover in a manner that is befitting a sacred moment.

Another way of setting the stage for love through the sacred senses of taste and smell is to prepare a small plate of delicious, romantic foods. Fresh fruit, chocolate, a small special treat, or a favorite wine can awaken the senses, heighten openness, and remind the lovers of even more delicious fruits to come. The Song of Songs makes liberal use of food in its imagery, referring to wine, honey, sweetmeats, nectar, and many other delicacies of the time.

Of course, kissing is the most prominent way the sense of taste can be employed by Infallible Lovers. As the lovers in the Song of Songs proclaim, "Your lips drip honey, my bride, sweetmeats and milk are under your tongue."

Take time to kiss each other, sweetly and gently at first and more passionately as things progress. Don't rush through this time together. Start with gentle kisses and light nibbles of each other's lips before moving to French kissing. Taste each other's lips and mouth, and then taste each other's bodies. Feel free to heighten all of your lover's senses with your kisses of his or her whole body — neck, hands and fingers, chest/breasts, stomach, and so on. Follow the example of the bride in the Song of Songs (4:16), who exclaims, "Blow upon my garden that its perfumes may spread abroad. Let my lover come to his garden and eat its choice fruits." Like the lovers of Sacred Scripture, eat and drink of your love for one another.

There are those who will have questions about oral stimulation of the genitals. (I do not say "oral sex" because to many this implies stimulation to ejaculation, which is morally problematic.) As long as couples are mindful of the One Rule, according to which a man must climax inside the woman, Catholic teaching does not forbid the passionate kissing of the penis or the labia (outer and inner) and clitoris any more than it forbids passionately kissing any other part of the body. Many men and women find this practice to be a very pleasurable and emotionally meaningful act. Some speak of the deep intimacy and even honor they feel when they and their mate feel safe and open enough to kiss one another in this most intimate and private way.

Others object to orally stimulating the genitals for the same reasons that they object to certain permitted sexual positions, or anything that feels too erotic. Many women, especially, because they have been taught that only immoral women do "that sort of thing," fear that they will be objectified by their husbands. Many others, men and women, have a gut reaction that tells them this is unhygienic.

The bottom line, however, is that as long as the couple respects the One Rule, is using the Four Pleasure Principles to guide their discernment, observes a continuity to respect that flows from their day-to-day relationship and informs their sexual relationship, and maintains basic cleanliness and hygiene, oral stimulation of the genitals is every bit as moral, safe, and healthy as kissing any other part of the body. Though this can be a deeply emotionally charged issue for many couples, as far as the Church is concerned, this is a matter that falls squarely in the realm of prudential judgment (as opposed to moral principles). Couples should be careful to respect each other's feelings, to resist the temptation to place barriers to intimacy that even the Church does not see fit to impose, and to deal with each other charitably in discussing such sensitive matters.

Having examined the various ways a couple can engage their senses of taste and scent in preparing one another to celebrate the sacred mysteries of Holy Sex, let's look at some ways you and your mate can expand your capacity to love each other more fully through these senses.

Quiz

MAXIMIZING THE SENSES OF TASTE AND SMELL IN FOREPLAY

1. Using a scale from 1 (not at all important) to 5 (completely important), rate the following items according to how big a role each plays in helping you prepare for lovemaking.

His　Hers

☐　☐　Oral hygiene (brushing teeth, mouthwash, etc.).

☐　☐　Cleanliness (showering, grooming hair, shaving).

☐　☐　Perfume/cologne. Describe.

☐　☐　Scented candles or other room fragrances. Describe.

☐　☐　Romantic foods. Describe.

☐　☐　Kissing (lips and mouth). Describe favorite kinds of kissing.

☐　☐　Kissing (the body). Describe what you like.

☐　☐　Other 1. Describe.

☐　☐　Other 2. Describe.

2. Considering what you have read about the spirituality of sensuality and sexuality, describe why the things you indicated above are as important to you as they are. Try to go beyond statements such as "I like it" or "It feels good." Instead, try to describe what it *means* to you to have your spouse do those things for you or with you.

3. What do you think you might need to do to make sure you include these aspects of foreplay in your lovemaking? (Remember to use the Four Pleasure Principles to negotiate any conflict around these items.)

Sight

You are all-beautiful, my beloved, and there is no blemish in you.
How beautiful are your feet in sandals, O prince's daughter!
Your rounded thighs are like jewels, the handiwork of an artist.
Your navel is a round bowl that should never lack for mixed wine.
Your body is a heap of wheat encircled with lilies.
Your breasts are like twin fawns, the young of a gazelle.

(Song 4:7, 7:2–5)

The sense of sight enables lovers to perceive and receive each other at their best. Infallible Lovers know the importance of making love in a space that is as beautiful as possible, or at least clean and neat. They may use candlelight or low light so that they can see one another, literally and figuratively, in the most attractive light.

Some couples blanch at the idea of making love with the lights on at all. If you feel this way, prayerfully reflect on the Second Power of Holy Sex and the beauty of vulnerability. Assuming that your relationship is such that it is safe to be vulnerable to each other at all, by challenging this reluctance to be seen by your lover, you are challenging an unhealthy tendency to cling to shame in the presence of love. Pope John Paul II noted that before the Fall, Adam and Eve enjoyed an innocent love that allowed them to be naked without shame. While we can never achieve that degree of purity this side of heaven, couples can help each other learn to look upon each other with the perfect love that casts out fear of intimacy (1 John 4:18). Overcoming this hyperactive sense of bodily shame can become both a spiritually and relationally freeing exercise.

In addition to preparing an attractive space for your lovemaking and making it possible to see each other in your best light, give some thought to the role that lingerie and other attractive attire may play in your foreplay. Just as the celebrant of the sacrament of the Eucharist wears beautiful vestments to set apart what is common from what is extraordinary, Infallible Lovers should feel free to use those articles of clothing that help them feel as if they are setting themselves apart for the special celebration that is the incarnation of their love.

Some people think that such garments are somehow unwholesome. I have heard some spouses, especially women, say that even the thought of wearing sensual apparel intended to enhance the experience of lovemaking makes them feel like they are being asked to dress or act like "common whores." This is truly unfortunate. A woman (or a man) degrades herself by using her body in the wrong way, at inappropriate times, in inappropriate contexts, with inappropriate people. This is what makes the behavior of a promiscuous person or a porn star sinful and unacceptable, *not* the clothes he or she is or is not wearing. You might as well say that since those unfortunate women are engaging in eroticism on a bed or in a house, you will never make love to your spouse in a bed or in your home. To blame the sensual trappings for the sinful behavior is to make the Puritan mistake of confusing glamour with the evil that hides behind it.

If you struggle with the fear of using certain articles of clothing, sexual positions, or other items that may enhance your sexual pleasure, especially because you know that they're often used in unwholesome ways by unchaste people, I encourage you to reflect on Romans 14 and 1 Corinthians 8. There, St. Paul addresses the problem early Christians had with eating meat that was sacrificed at a pagan temple and then sold at market. St. Paul's ruling? Meat that is dedicated to Zeus (or whomever), is still meat that was made by God, and as long as a Christian thanks God, and not Zeus (or whomever) for it, then the Christian is doing nothing wrong. Paul asserts that things are not bad in and of themselves. Rather, the improper use of things is bad. Furthermore, the abuse of an item by some does not negate the use of that item by all.

Bottom line? If you make some sexual thing more important than your partner, or only want to engage in some act or manner of dress because you watched it on your favorite porn video, then yes, Houston, we have a problem. But assuming you and your mate are approaching each other as Infallible Lovers, then as Paul says, "To the pure, all things are pure" (Tit. 1:15). In sum, there is nothing objectively wrong with almost any type of sensual attire as long as its use respects the spirit of the Four Pleasure Principles.

There is one other common objection to lingerie and attractive bedroom attire that I would like to address but has nothing to do with morality. Some people (and this applies to both men and women) object to dressing attractively in anticipation of lovemaking because they feel like they're being "fake." They resent feeling as if "they're not good enough just the way they are." While it is good to be wanted just for who you are, this line of thinking makes no sense at all. After all, if you really feel this way, why would you ever get dressed up for anything? Why not show up at Mass, a formal banquet, or a wedding feast, in a ratty old T-shirt and sweats because they're comfy and you don't care to "pretend to be someone you are not"?

While clothes are not the most important thing and you should be made to feel perfectly welcome by the people at Mass — or any of those other places — in your ratty T-shirt or sweats, that's not really the point. We dress well for certain occasions so that we can make an attractive gift of ourselves to others. We try to dress attractively at Mass so that we can make as fine a gift of ourselves to the Lord as possible. We dress for the banquet to honor the host and the dignity of the occasion. We dress for the concert to honor the performers and acknowledge the dignity of their art. In the same way, lovers should feel free to dress as attractively as they can for each other in order to make as fine a gift of themselves to each other as possible and to give honor to the dignity of the art of their love. Of course, it could also be said that there is nothing so attractive as each lover's naked body. I am not spending so much time on the question of sexual attire because it is a *necessary* part of foreplay. Far from it. Rather I am addressing it because there seems to be so much confusion and erroneous suspicion about its use. Suffice it to say, as long as a couple is being mindful of the Four Pleasure Principles, they may feel free to wear *or not wear* just about whatever they like in their attempt to present themselves as the most beautiful and handsome gift they can be to each other.

Take a moment to answer the following questions about the visual aspects of foreplay that matter most to you.

Quiz
MAXIMIZING THE VISUAL SENSE IN FOREPLAY

1. Using a scale from 1 (not at all important) to 5 (completely important), rate the following items according to how big a role each plays in helping you prepare for lovemaking.

His	Hers	
☐	☐	A neat and clean room.
☐	☐	Attractive lighting (candles, soft lights).
☐	☐	A romantic setting. Describe.
☐	☐	Lingerie or other attractive attire. Describe.
☐	☐	Other 1. Describe.
☐	☐	Other 2. Describe.

2. Considering what you have read about the spirituality of sensuality and sexuality, describe why the things you indicated above are as important to you as they are. Be specific.

3. What do you think you might need to do to make sure you include these aspects of foreplay in your lovemaking? (Remember to use the Four Pleasure Principles to negotiate any conflicts.)

Hearing

Hark! my lover — here he comes springing across the mountains, leaping across the hills. (Songs 2:8)

Your sense of hearing is of utmost importance in lovemaking because it helps root you in the moment, communicate your likes and dislikes, and affirm your lover's ability to please you.

Most people's heads are swimming at the end of the day from all the noise of the business of their lives. What didn't I get done today? Where do I have to take the kids tomorrow? What was that appointment I had tomorrow? Appropriate music (or in some cases, intentional silence), tender words, and helpful indicators that you are pleasing your mate (in the form of either verbal direction or nonverbal sounds of pleasure) quiet all the noise in your head and help you focus on being fully present to your partner. Your sense of hearing helps you center in on your lover in the here and now.

Some people feel awkward sharing tender words or making sounds that let their mate know their mate is pleasing them. It makes them feel self-conscious. Others find it distracting. For those couples who find it distracting, and by mutual agreement prefer to minimize any auditory distractions, there is certainly no obligation to become more verbal or expressive during foreplay and lovemaking. But those who object to being more verbally expressive on the grounds that it feels self-conscious or vaguely "wrong" — especially over the requests of your lover to be more expressive — should try to work through the process described in the Four Pleasure Principles section (pp. 192ff.). Just as there is nothing objectively wrong with making yourself look as attractive and enticing as possible, there is nothing objectively wrong with being more verbally expressive. In fact, you could make the argument that it's *virtuous* to do so. How? If your sense of hearing roots you in the here and now during lovemaking, by refusing to be more verbally expressive, you may be choosing to stay somewhere else in your head where you are not as safe and loved as you are now in the arms of your lover. Assuming that you're being mindful of the Four Pleasure Principles, your spouse deserves all of you, and your mate will feel rightfully offended if you hold back.

Again, though, I'm not suggesting that a couple must put on a concert. There is no need to moan and shout so that it can be heard for miles around. Nor am I suggesting that any sound is necessary at all. It certainly is not. I'm simply pointing out that the more sensual the experience of lovemaking is, the easier it is for the body to do the job God gave it to do — namely, to render visible (able to be perceived by the senses) that which is invisible (the love between the couple). You both should feel free to make whatever sounds, or enjoy whatever sounds, draw you closer to each other.

One other issue we should deal with in our discussion of the sense of hearing is that of sharing your fantasies with one another. Fantasies involving sinful acts (like swinging, or sex with multiple partners, or humiliating acts) may require counseling to sort out. These can be as problematic as they are common, and they warrant special attention because they are degrading to the person and the couple. Exploring unhealthy or sinful fantasies in counseling, rather than being a source of condemnation, can reveal important paths to greater personal or relational health. We'll discuss more about knowing when to seek professional help in chapter 22.

Leaving aside the issue of fantasies involving objectively degrading acts, let's briefly discuss the role of sharing more benign fantasies as part of foreplay. Engaging in playful, erotic storytelling, discussing intimate details of how you might wish to please each other, even some degree of role-playing can be perfectly acceptable. By their very nature, fantasies involve pushing the boundaries of the lover's comfort zones, and this can be good or bad, depending upon the specific circumstances. Generally, exploring fantasies can be a safe way to both heighten desire in the moment and set up future discussions about how Infallible Lovers can be more pleasing to one another. But do remember the Pleasure Principles that refer to both the need for continuity between your daily relationship and your sexual relationship, *and* the need to make sure that celebrating love — not creating an erotic event — is the real point of your lovemaking. If you are playful with each other during the day and you share fantasies that emphasize and increase this sense of playfulness in the bedroom, this can be delightful. But if you can be aroused only when your mate is pretending to be someone else, or when you are pretending to be with someone else, fantasy ceases to be healthy. (Once again, for more complicated issues related to morally questionable or personally offensive fantasies, please see chapter 22.)

Regardless of the question of sharing fantasies, increasing your experience of your sense of hearing in the bedroom by being more vocal and verbal during lovemaking can be a very important way of orienting yourself to the present and sharing your body, your self, and your innermost thoughts more completely with your spouse.

In light of this, take a moment to answer the following questions about the auditory aspects of foreplay that matter most to you.

Quiz
MAXIMIZING THE AUDITORY SENSE
IN FOREPLAY

1. Using a scale from 1 (not at all important) to 5 (completely important), rate the following items according to how big a role each plays in helping you prepare for lovemaking.

His   Hers

☐   ☐   Romantic music. Describe.

☐   ☐   Speaking tender words of love. Give examples.

☐   ☐   Giving and receiving direct verbal feedback about what does and does not feel good to your partner. Give examples.

☐   ☐   Hearing your partner make sounds (sighs, moans, giggles, etc.) that let you know that what you are doing is pleasing to your mate.

☐   ☐   Telling each other romantic or erotic fantasies or stories.

☐ ☐ Other 1. Describe.

☐ ☐ Other 2. Describe.

2. Considering what you have read about the spirituality of sensuality and sexuality, describe why the things you indicated above are as important to you as they are. Be specific.

3. What do you think you might need to do to make sure you include these aspects of foreplay in your lovemaking? (Remember to use the Four Pleasure Principles to negotiate any conflict.)

Touch

Your very figure is like a palm tree, your breasts are like clusters. I said: I will climb the palm tree, I will take hold of its branches. Now let your breasts be like clusters of the vine and the fragrance of your breath like apples, and your mouth like an excellent wine — that flows smoothly for my lover, spreading over the lips and the teeth. (Song 7:8–10)

Touch is perhaps the most obvious of the senses that come into play during foreplay and lovemaking, but in some ways it is the most deceptive. Too many couples think that because they are touching each other — and especially because they are touching each other's genitals — they are engaging in foreplay. This is really not the case.

Touch is the way that lovers announce to each other "I am present *for* you. I am making myself a present *to* you." Imagine for a moment someone jumping out at you and screaming "TA DA!" through a bullhorn. This is the equivalent of rushing right to groping each other's genitals in the name of foreplay.

Let's start over now. This time, imagine that you are awaiting your lover's return home from work. Suddenly, you hear the distant sounds of your lover's car coming down the street, pulling into the driveway. Now your lover's feet are on the front steps, at the door, in the house, walking to the bedroom. Each new sound announces, "I am coming for you. I love you. I can't wait to rediscover you." This is what touch should be like in foreplay — a gentle, slowly building drumbeat that announces your presence to each other's bodies more and more intently until you are each excitedly anticipating the consummation of your love.

Having described these two scenarios, which do you think, generally speaking, is more appealing? Oh, sure, the occasional surprise party is wonderful. On those nights when you already feel so close to each other and don't have a lot of time, allowing your bodies to jump out and shout "TA DA!" is perfectly acceptable, but if your circumstances allow you to do more, then why not do more?

Try to begin with the softest and gentlest touching you can. Linger. Recall the suggestion that "half as fast can feel twice as good." Try to focus on every part of your lover's body. Caress your lover's face. Kiss your lover's hands. Massage each other's neck and back. Intentionally avoid touching each other's genitals at first. As your kissing becomes more passionate, slowly move nearer and nearer to touching each other more intimately. Build the tension. Let each touch slowly reveal to your mate that you are approaching, slowly, nearer and nearer, readying each other to receive all you each have to offer one another. Learn to read each other's physical, verbal, and nonverbal cues. Even when a lover is not being intentionally expressive, he or she reveals certain subtle signs that pleasure and anticipation are increasing. By acquainting yourself with your lover's unique signs of arousal, you can pace your touch so that you gently and passionately guide each other across the bridge that joins intimate partnership to sexual intimacy. (See also the Harmonization Exercise, p. 255).

Marital Aids

Before wrapping up this section on touch, we should briefly touch on the matter of marital aids — in particular, devices such as vibrators and related items. Some couples find these devices especially useful — either during foreplay or as part of intercourse — in cases when the woman risks becoming frustrated because her husband has climaxed but she has not. Strictly speaking, there is nothing in Church teaching that forbids the use of marital aids in this manner, as long as they are not used by one spouse for masturbatory purposes and, pastorally speaking, the couple is mindful to use the Four Pleasure Principles in discerning the proper use of these devices. Even so, I've found that too many couples use these as stand-ins for real intimacy and communication and can come to rely too heavily upon them in their sexual relationship. This is problematic, because it means that the couple's capacity for sexual pleasure is not really rooted in their intimacy. Rather, sexual pleasure becomes too closely linked to the device the couple is using. The ultimate goal for the couple should be learning to do directly for each other what they previously relied on the marital aid to help them achieve — not to use the aid as a substitute for intimacy or communication. Remember, the point of lovemaking is to celebrate love. It is not about requiring something other than the couple to be present in order for the couple to be happy. Anything the couple does or uses in their lovemaking must be secondary to their own ability to love and please each other. Keeping all this in mind, a couple is free to use anything that *enhances* their ability to love each other, does not violate the One Rule, and is mindful of the Four Pleasure Principles. Couples must discern for themselves what this means regarding the use of most marital aids.

Quiz
MAXIMIZING THE SENSE OF TOUCH IN FOREPLAY

Take a moment to examine the ways you can more effectively use the sense of touch in foreplay.

1. Using a scale from 1 (not at all important) to 5 (completely important), rate the following items according to how large a role each plays in helping you prepare for lovemaking.

His   Hers

☐   ☐   Light kissing.

☐   ☐   French kissing.

☐	☐	Backrubs/massage.
☐	☐	Light scratching.
☐	☐	Other 1. Describe.
☐	☐	Other 2. Describe.

2. Considering what you have read about the spirituality of sensuality and sexuality, describe why the things you indicated above are as important to you as they are. Be specific.

3. What do you think you might need to do to make sure you include these aspects of foreplay in your lovemaking? (Remember to use the Four Pleasure Principles to negotiate any conflicts.)

4. Take a moment to identify the verbal and nonverbal signs your spouse gives you that let you know when it is time to move from less intimate touching to more intimate touching. If you aren't sure, ask your mate. For more help, refer to the Harmonization Exercise in our discussion on intercourse (p. 255). In what ways could your spouse make it clearer to you when he or she is ready to transition from lighter touching to more intimate touching?

The Stage Is Set

In this chapter, we have examined the spiritual and psychological significance of foreplay and explored practical ways that you can empower your body to more effectively do what God created it to do. Sensuality is an essential ingredient of spirituality. The more sensual your loving, the more able your bodies will be to make visible that which is invisible. That is, your bodies will be empowered to reveal yourselves to each other more fully and your love for each other more completely.

In the next chapter, we will look at lovemaking and the afterglow and how to celebrate the sacrament of Holy Sex to its fullest potential.

13 THE ANATOMY OF INFALLIBLE LOVING: THE GOOD STUFF

Indeed, the very words, "I take you as my wife — my husband..." can be fulfilled only by means of conjugal intercourse.

— Pope John Paul II

efore we begin, I have a little announcement. *Ahem.*

I imagine some curious readers and bookstore flippers (you know who you are) might jump ahead to this chapter because they want to get to the good stuff and see what I have to say about "doing the deed." If you're one of those readers, all I can say is if you approach sex like you're approaching this book — all in a rush to get to the big finish — no wonder you need help! As Monty Python said in *The Meaning of Life*, "Let's not go stampeding toward the clitoris, shall we?" I'll be sure to offer up a rosary for you. Make that two. Now, kindly flip back to page 1 and begin at the beginning. You've got a lot to learn before you're ready for this.

To the rest of you patient and thoughtful readers who have made the long journey with me to this point, I say, "Welcome."

This chapter will simply not have the same impact for anyone who has not been along for the whole ride. Unless you have learned the tools for distinguishing Holy Sex from eroticism and discovered everything we have discussed about what it really takes to become an Infallible Lover, you won't be able to appreciate what this chapter has to offer. But if you've been working on all the skills we have explored throughout the book, you'll be ready to go deeper into the sacred mystery that is Holy Sex.

In the course of the next few pages, I'm going to provide some basic information on the spirituality of intercourse that builds upon everything we've discussed already. Next, we'll review some practical information about sexual positions. Finally, we'll examine how your sexual relationship can and should lead you to a deeper experience of love in your day-to-day relationship.

TRANSITIONING TO INTERCOURSE

In the last chapter, we explored the spiritual, psychological, and relational significance of foreplay and suggested many ways that Infallible Lovers could enable their bodies to more completely and passionately do what they were created to do — render visible that which is invisible (your love for each other). Through sensual foreplay, rooted in a profound respect for each other and the sacramental and incarnational dimensions of your sexual love, you have set the stage by awakening the senses and enkindling the fire of an eros that can empower you to rise up toward the Divine. Now it's time to discover how to let that warm, small fire turn into a blaze that consumes you and your lover and prepares you to melt into the light and heat of God's own love for each of you.

THE MIND-BLOWING SPIRITUALITY OF INTERCOURSE

In earlier chapters, we have made much of St. Paul's assertion in Ephesians 5:32 that the union between man and woman is a sign of Christ's union with his bride, the Church. In his writings on the Theology of the Body, Pope John Paul II observed that all of salvation history reveals that God enters into the world as the bridegroom and all of creation receives him as the bride. This nuptial imagery is the most basic and profound way we can illustrate the nature of the passionate, total, and *reciprocal* union God desires with each and every one of us.

I emphasized the word "reciprocal," because God doesn't just want us to lie back and be loved by him. True, he wants us to abandon ourselves and surrender totally to him, but he challenges us to an active abandonment and an intentional surrender. In other words, he wants us to love him in return. God doesn't offer himself to us and invite us to respond because he needs us in any way. He is complete and whole all by himself. He does this because he *chooses* us to be his intimate partners despite his lack of need for anything. "The Son of man became man so that men might become gods" (CCC no. 460).

This is a mind-blowing concept, but one way we can begin to wrap our heads around it is to place it in the context of Holy Sex, which Catholics believe was created by God to image the nature of his own relationship with us. What does this mean? In healthy relationships, lovers do not "need" each other in the sense that an addict needs his fix. Even though they are capable of a certain level of completeness on their own, they *choose* each other, and they choose to give and receive each other fully in a free, fruitful, and faithful covenant of love. In a similar way, God, who has no need of us, *chooses* us to be his partners anyway and goes to great lengths to give himself totally to us. Moreover, he invites us to do the same, creating a free, fruitful, and faithful union between heaven and earth.

Because of the way God made our bodies, masculinity is essentially *donative* (i.e., "giving") in nature and femininity is essentially *receptive* ("receiving") in nature. In other words, God has made our bodies so that in lovemaking, the man enters into the woman and the woman receives the man. But this isn't the end of the story. In giving himself, the man also receives the woman, and in receiving the man, the woman gives herself to him. In Holy Sex, the man isn't just some sexual aggressor and the woman some passive recipient who lies back, grits her teeth, and "thinks of the Vatican." Rather, Pope John Paul II argued that what I call Holy Sex involves "interpenetration" whereby man and woman totally give themselves to each other and receive each other totally in return. As Christopher West writes of this active, reciprocal union in *The Theology of the Body Explained*:

> *The male, by virtue of the specific nuptial dynamism of his body, is disposed toward giving or initiating the gift. The female, by virtue of the specific nuptial dynamism of her body, is disposed toward accepting or receiving*

the gift. Nonetheless, "giving" does not belong exclusively to the male and "receiving" does not belong exclusively to the female. They interpenetrate so that in giving the male receives and in receiving the female gives.

In a similar way, God, the divine bridegroom, enters into creation — and creation receives his love. But we are not just passive recipients of God's love. He invites us into intimate partnership whereby we give ourselves as deeply and profoundly as we are receiving him. God's love for humankind, and our love for God, is an active, passionate love that demands total receptivity *and* total self-gift.

There is, of course, a profound philosophical and theological significance to all of this that goes beyond the scope of this book. What it means for our more practical purposes is that in order for a man and woman to fully *experience* the power of Holy Sex as a sign of God's union with us, both the man and woman must be fully engaged in their entire relationship, including their sexual relationship. Both must actively challenge themselves to seek more and deeper ways to give to and receive from each other every moment of every day. This is most especially highlighted in the sexual interplay between husband and wife. Holy Sex cannot occur in situations where the husband is pursuing a totally passive and unreceptive or resistant wife. Nor can it occur in situations where the husband is unwilling to *receive* the woman's heart and mind and soul as well as her body.

When a man and a woman are both actively engaged as Infallible Lovers — each giving to and receiving from one another as fully as possible in every area of their lives — then they begin to reveal, on a physical level, the kind of love and commitment God invites them to share with him. Then can their bodies make visible what is invisible. It is at that point that Holy Sex begins to manifest its full spiritual potential.

Is there anything holding you back from making this free and total commitment to "interpenetration" with your mate?

Quiz
HOW ENGAGED ARE YOU?

The following statements will help you evaluate the level of "inter-penetration" you experience specifically in your sexual relationship. On a scale of 1 (Completely False) to 5 (Completely True), rate the following statements.

His Hers

☐ ☐ 1. I am a full and active participant in lovemaking with my spouse.

☐ ☐ 2. I actively think about our sexual relationship and the ways I can give myself more fully to my spouse during lovemaking.

☐ ☐ 3. I regularly ask my spouse to tell me what he or she needs in and from our sexual relationship.

☐ ☐ 4. When my spouse tells me what he or she needs in and from our sexual relationship, I work hard to remember and incorporate what I hear.

☐ ☐ 5. I eagerly try to learn how I can give more of myself to my partner in our sexual relationship.

☐ ☐ 6. I am playful during lovemaking. I enjoy trying new things and look for ways to increase our repertoire of ways to be physically present to one another.

☐ ☐ 7. I look forward to sex and often tell my mate how eagerly I anticipate the next time we can be sexually intimate.

☐ ☐ 8. Assuming that my mate is not asking to do anything that is morally illicit, I receive my mate's suggestions during lovemaking warmly and with an open mind and heart.

☐ ☐ 9. I am comfortable initiating sex and making my needs known during lovemaking.

☐ ☐ 10. When my spouse and I have disagreements about our sexual relationship, I willingly commit time and energy to working through those issues with my partner.

This quiz is not meant to be scored. It is meant to give you an opportunity to reflect on the ways you can be more open to giving yourselves to each other in your sexual relationship. Discuss the following:

1. In those areas where you find yourself resisting the call to be more giving or more receptive, what percentage of this withholding is due to personal discomfort with sexuality and what percentage to concerns about your relationship?

_____ percent personal struggles vs. _____ percent relationship concerns

Example:

    30 percent personal concerns vs. 70 percent relationship concerns

2. If you attributed any percentage of your tendency to hold back in your sexual relationship to personal concerns, what are those concerns?

3. What are the relationship concerns?

4. Check the resources you think could be most helpful to you in overcoming these issues.

    _____ Couple Prayer

    _____ Counseling

    _____ Arguing Skills

    _____ Medical Evaluation

    _____ Marriage Retreat

    _____ Employing the Four Pleasure Principles (p. 192)

    _____ Improving Marital Rituals and Routines (p. 210)

    _____ Marital Checkup Exercise (p. 213)

    _____ Lovelist Exercise (p. 214)

    _____ Others. Describe.

5. Identify specific steps that will help you access these resources. (Examples: "Call diocese to find out about marriage retreat." "Make doctor's appt." "Call Pastoral Solutions Institute for counseling or seek local referral.")

Now that we've established the importance of both the husband and wife being actively engaged in intercourse in order to enjoy the full sensual, spiritual, and psychological fruit of the experience, let's talk about the experience itself.

It can be a challenge for faithful couples to find practical resources they can use to learn more about intercourse. In light of this, I would like to present some basic information on sexual positions and give you the opportunity to discuss with your beloved the ways you can create as sensual, and in turn as spiritual, an encounter as possible.

LEARNING FROM THE WOMAN'S BODY

As we consider lovemaking itself, it is important, especially for a man, to learn to listen to what his wife's body tells him about the best ways to please her. Simply put, what is pleasing to a woman today, sexually speaking, may not feel good at all tomorrow. This can be extraordinarily frustrating for husbands who often feel that their wives are simply being intentionally difficult and refusing to be pleased. Many husbands I counsel wish their wives could just give them a script that they could follow. "Press this. Rub that. Kaboom! Great Sex." For that matter, many women I counsel who are not familiar with their bodies feel guilty or frustrated because they don't understand why they feel as they do and why it's so difficult to articulate their needs to their husband. Alternatively, a woman may feel that her husband is a clumsy oaf for just not getting it.

There is no simple script a man and woman can use to automatically have an incredible sexual experience every time. Each time will be a little different because a woman's body is actually a little different every time she makes love. As we began to discover in the chapter on NFP, the degree of lubrication, the sensitivity of genital nerve-endings and tenderness of the labia, as well as the actual structure of the vagina and position of the cervix change from day to day based on where a woman is in her cycle. Pleasing a woman can sometimes be so frustrating for a man because he feels like he is shooting at a moving target — which, in fact, he literally is. One of the practical reasons I spend so much of the book focusing on relationship, relationship, relationship is because if you haven't established a high level of intimacy, communication, and vulnerability in your day-to-day relationship, you will never achieve the degree of humility, and your spouse will never achieve the degree of openness, you both need to communicate what will give you both the most pleasure today.

To give you and your spouse the opportunity to understand each other a little better, let's examine how the stages of a woman's cycle relate to sexual pleasure.

Phase I Loving

In the most general terms, a woman will probably feel the most tender and sensitive during Phase I of her cycle (the time from menstruation to the beginning of the pre-ovulatory phase — usually about the first six to ten days or so of her cycle). Many couples prefer not to make love at all during Phase I because of concerns about the messiness of her period or — if her menstrual flow has stopped — the soreness she experiences following menstruation. However, if a couple wishes to make love during Phase I, they are certainly permitted to. Unlike Orthodox Jews, who object to intercourse during Phase I because of ritual impurity, Christians have no moral objections to intercourse during the entire first phase of the woman's cycle if they are so inclined. Assuming proper hormonal function, a woman's menstrual flow should not normally last more than four or five days. Longer periods may indicate problems (hypothyroidism is most common) that may be corrected with nutritional interventions (see *Fertility, Cycles, and Nutrition* by Marilyn Shannon) or via consultation with a physician trained in Natural Procreative Technology (NaPro Technology).

A husband should definitely be aware that his wife's body will most likely be very sensitive and tender during this time. If a couple wishes to be intimate during Phase I, husbands and wives should proceed gently at first, taking more time with foreplay than they might otherwise take (focusing more on touching and kissing other parts of the body besides the breasts and genitals, which can be quite tender), and choosing sexual positions that do not favor the deepest penetration possible at first. Regarding this latter point, couples may want to focus on positions that allow the woman to control the depth of penetration (such as the woman on top or positions that involve the couple sitting and facing each other), giving her the ability to make immediate adjustments in case she begins to feel at all uncomfortable.

These are, of course, no strict rules. It's up to the couple to communicate about what feels good and at what point during lovemaking, but generally speaking, sex during Phase I will at least *begin* as a gentler affair, and husbands should not expect their wives to be in their most energetic or acrobatic place.

Phase II Loving

During Phase II of a woman's cycle (the fertile phase, lasting about ten days or so), the woman experiences a rush of hormones that tend to make her much more aroused. Her levels of vaginal lubrication increase dramatically, and her cervix opens and rises to a higher position in the vagina. Generally speaking, couples who are not abstaining for purposes of avoiding pregnancy during this phase will find that this is a wonderful time for more playful sexual expression and experimentation. Although couples should still take time to set the stage for intercourse with adequate foreplay as we discussed in the last chapter, there is usually less of a physiological need for extended foreplay during this phase of the woman's cycle because the lubrication and arousal levels of the woman are already higher at this point than at any other time of the month.

During Phase II, couples may wish to experiment with new positions, and emphasize sexual positions that allow deeper penetration (such as the missionary position and variations on it, the man entering from behind the woman, or woman-on-top). Generally speaking, a woman will physiologically be at her most energetic and sexually aroused point during this phase, and she will often be more open to new suggestions. Once again, however, communication is key here. Couples should continue to be open with each other about what feels best for them and should avoid turning lovemaking into a test or task that they can pass or fail. Remember, the point of lovemaking is celebrating love, not staging an experience. Focus on loving each other and on your partner to guide you well.

Phase III Loving

Phase III of a woman's cycle (beginning a few days after ovulation and lasting until the first day of her period — about ten days or so) is called the "luteal phase," and it is brought on by an increase in the woman's progesterone levels. This causes a lessening of vaginal lubrication, the lowering, closing, and hardening of the cervix in the vagina, and a relative decrease in the woman's level of physiological arousal. Later in the luteal phase, hormonal shifts may bring on what is commonly referred to as PMS. Couples making love in this phase would do well to follow similar recommendations as I made previously with regard to lovemaking during Phase I. That is, employ extended foreplay and sexual positions favoring more shallow penetration at first, and then move to positions allowing deeper penetration later as lubrication and arousal levels allow. Some couples may find the use of personal lubricants helpful for compensating for the woman's drop in natural lubrication during this phase.

Arousal, Intimacy, and Phase III

Couples can sometimes become frustrated during Phase III because of the drop in hormonal arousal that occurs with the build-up of progesterone in the system. While some nutritional or NaPro Technology interventions may be helpful, the most important thing is for a couple to root their sexual relationship in *intimacy*, not just physiological arousal. We will discuss this further in the chapter addressing low sexual desire, but for now we note that relying on physiological arousal alone to be the catalyst for sexual intimacy is an all too common mistake that can doom lovemaking.

Lesser lovers think of sex as "scratching an itch." If they don't feel aroused, then they aren't "in the mood," and they tend to be disinclined to make love. Women, incidentally, are as likely to be arousal-driven as men with regard to their sexual desire. The difference is that men are always fertile and therefore always physiologically aroused (or arousable), while women are fertile only for a few days a month and therefore experience their greatest degree of physiological arousal periodically. If a couple bases their sexual relationship on arousal alone, then what most often happens is that the man becomes the sexual pursuer and the woman is put in the position of constantly saying that she "just doesn't feel like it tonight."

Infallible Lovers, however, know that arousal is a less important driver of sexual intercourse than intimacy. Arousal, being primarily a physiological phenomenon, is susceptible to physiological factors like exhaustion, stress, illness, and even accommodation (getting used to somebody). Because of this, Infallible Lovers know that while arousal itself is desirable, it is intimacy that will propel a couple to seek the comfort of each other's arms even when they are tired, stressed, sick, or frazzled. Without stretching themselves to grow in the virtues we identified in chapter 3 as essential for becoming an Infallible Lover, and without investing the time and energy needed for creating the kind of friendship, safety, vulnerability, and partnership upon which intimacy relies, a couple has only arousal to count on, and arousal cannot be reliably counted on.

We will revisit this theme in a later chapter. Suffice it to say that lovemaking at all times must be driven by the intimacy a couple shares in their entire relationship. Regardless of the particular phase a couple is in, they will need to be sensitive to each other, and they will need to respect what the woman's body is telling them about how they can best approach each other in order to experience a fully satisfying sexual relationship.

REVIEWING YOUR SEXUAL REPERTOIRE: POSITIONS AND MORE

Now that you know a bit about how to read what your bodies say about how to approach each other during lovemaking, let's review some of the sexual positions that make up the basic sexual repertoire. Couples often argue about which sexual positions to use. As we discussed in our chapter on pleasure, almost anything that respects the One Rule (in short, the man must climax inside the woman) and is mindful of the Four Pleasure Principles is absolutely permissible. Let's recap those principles here.

1. There should be continuity between your daily relationship and your sexual relationship.

2. While you should never be afraid to explore all the permitted pleasures, you should never be tempted to see each other merely as givers and receivers of pleasure. You must always respect the dignity of each other as persons.

3. Any sexual positions, items, articles of clothing, manners of speech, or playful actions used to help you achieve the fullness of sexual pleasure should be used in a manner that helps you and your beloved draw closer to each other, not to the thing. Things should never become the primary point of the sexual relationship. Rather, they should be seen as the means you employ to experience the fullness of each other's love.

4. While a lover's comfort zones should not be the final arbiter in sexual disputes, feelings related to comfort zones must be respected. A lover's discomfort is reason enough to delay participating in some sensual activity, even if it is not enough to rule out entirely future participation in that activity. The couple should continue to evaluate all permitted pleasures in the light of the relationship and in a spirit of prayer.

As long as a couple is respectful of the One Rule and the Four Pleasure Principles, Infallible Lovers should feel free to enjoy all of the positions described over the following pages as well as the many that we don't have room to discuss. Assuming the couple is mindful of the One Rule, the question of sexual positions is a prudential matter that each couple must freely discern for themselves in a spirit of love and charity.

Man-on-Top Positions

This is commonly referred to as the missionary position, although the popular notion that it was the only position permitted by missionaries is an urban legend. Another NACWATC myth bites the dust.

Kinsey reported that over 90 percent of couples use man-on-top positions most often and with good reason since they are intimate, versatile, and simple to achieve. The man-on-top positions allow for deep penetration and are considered best for achieving pregnancy, because they allow the vagina to retain more semen upon the completion of intercourse. Likewise, man-on-top positions are very intimate positions. They are good for those couples who want to be able to kiss and caress each other as well as meet each other's gaze while making love.

To achieve the basic man-on-top position, a woman will lie on her back with her legs open. The man will then either lie directly on top of her, or he can support his weight with his arms. Either the man or the woman can then guide the penis into the vagina. Once the husband has entered his wife, he basically controls the rhythm and depth of thrusting, taking the role of active-giver to the woman's role as active-receiver. Because the man is in control of lovemaking in the man-on-top family of positions, he should be careful to take his cues from the woman's response to him rather than his own level of arousal. Even so, in her role as active-receiver, the woman can increase the depth of penetration by opening her legs wider, or raising her knees to her chest and/or resting her legs on her husband's shoulders — feet behind his head — for the deepest degree of penetration. For those couples who wish to allow the vagina to more tightly grip the penis, the woman may bring both legs to rest on her husband's left or right shoulder, crossing her ankles. This allows the man to continue to thrust easily while tightening the vaginal walls around the penis.

The woman can also increase her level of clitoral stimulation by pressing herself against her husband while he thrusts. The clitoris, of course, is a small external female sex organ comprised of several thousand — upward of ten thousand — tightly packed nerves at the top tip of the inner labia that, like a tiny penis, becomes engorged with arousal — though it does not ejaculate — and can play an important role in sexual pleasure. In her role as active-receiver, it is important that the woman know how to cooperate with her husband so that both may achieve all the pleasure God intends for the couple from the marital act.

Additionally, it can sometimes be helpful for a woman to place a pillow behind the small of her back to raise her pelvis so that the couple can achieve the greatest level of genital contact with the greatest degree of comfort for both. Another variation on this position involves the woman lying on the edge of the bed (or other raised surface such as a table or chair) with the man standing between her legs and in front of the woman.

Woman-on-Top Positions

Woman-on-top positions are good for those times when the woman wishes to control the depth of penetration and the rhythm of thrusting. Examples might include those times of her cycle when she is more tender, in which case she might prefer gentler and more shallow penetration, or those times when she is especially aroused and wants to feel her husband most deeply. This position can be good for Phase III lovemaking because it allows the woman to vary the depth of penetration as her lubrication and arousal increases.

Some couples believe that only aggressive women like to be on top, but this is not the case at all. Infallible Lovers know that Holy Sex is never about power politics. Holy Sex is about being willing to use whatever permitted means are available to a couple to achieve the fullness of their sexual experience — both sensually and spiritually.

The basic woman-on-top position is achieved when a man lies on his back and the woman straddles him, guiding his penis inside of her. Intercourse may then continue with the woman either in a kneeling position, or the woman lying on top of the man with her legs resting on the outside of his. The woman can also control clitoral stimulation by shifting forward a bit and rubbing her groin against the man while she moves on top of him. To stimulate her G-Spot (a bundle of sensitive nerves located toward the front of the vagina under the pelvic bone) the woman, in a kneeling position facing her husband, can lean back, putting her arms behind her while continuing to straddle her husband. Some women find G-spot stimulation highly pleasurable; others don't. G-spot stimulation is not necessary for achieving orgasm, and the woman should not feel any pressure to experience it, or frustration if she doesn't feel any difference.

Like with the man-on-top positions, the basic woman-on-top positions are very intimate and romantic, allowing the couple to kiss and look into each other's eyes while they make love. Another variation on this position can also be pleasing to some couples, however. This is when the woman straddles the man while facing away from him, then, resting on her arms and legs with his penis inside her, she guides the rhythm of thrusting while remaining on all fours. While this position is, in some ways, less romantic than the basic woman-on-top position, there are other benefits to the man and woman. Some men, especially men who are more visual, find the view of the wife moving up and down on the penis very erotic. For the woman, this angle of penetration moves the penis to the front of the vagina and may provide additional stimulation to the G-spot.

In all variations of the woman-on-top position, the woman is very much in the role of active-receiver and the man is very much in the role of receiving-giver. As such, the man, who is not able to move much, is placed in a more dependent position, being taken care of, while giving the woman an opportunity to take charge of the relationship. This dynamic allows couples to, in a sense, reverse roles, albeit in a way that does not diminish the masculinity of the man or the femininity of the woman. Some couples find this aspect of woman-on-top positions appealing, and others do not. St. Augustine's dictum applies, "In necessary things unity, in doubtful matters freedom, in all things charity." Each couple is free to make up their own mind about what works for them.

Man-from-Behind Positions*

Man-from-behind positions allow for very deep penetration and vigorous thrusting. This can be very exciting for the woman who has sufficient lubrication and arousal, especially if her cervix is higher up in the vaginal canal. For some women, however, these positions can be painful, especially when the cervix is lower in the vagina since penetration is so deep.

Man-from-behind positions can be achieved in two primary ways. The woman may either get on her hands and knees, raising her hips, while the man kneels behind her, or the woman may lean over an object (like a bed, table, or chair) while the man positions himself behind her. From this position, the man may fondle the woman's breasts or stimulate her clitoris manually while thrusting from behind. This can be highly pleasurable — physically and psychologically — for the woman who especially enjoys being in the role of active-receiver.

As with woman-on-top positions, some couples object to those positions in which the man enters the woman from behind because it implies submission or seems animalistic. Once again, although every couple is free to decide what they are comfortable with, there is nothing in Catholic teaching that forbids man-from-behind positions.

Likewise, assuming that the couple's day-to-day relationship is loving, intimate, respectful, and deeply humane, there is nothing objectively demeaning or animalistic about these positions and many couples find them both pleasurable and emotionally edifying exactly because this position

---

*Man-from-behind positions should not be confused with anal sex. That said, as Christopher West has noted in his book *Good News about Sex and Marriage,* there is nothing technically forbidding a couple from engaging in anal penetration as part of foreplay (remember, the man must ultimately climax inside the woman). However, because there are many bacteria in the anus, a couple should never move from anal penetration to vaginal intercourse without the man first washing his penis thoroughly, although antibacterial soap can cause irritation to sensitive vaginal tissue. For this reason, most secular sex therapists recommend the use of a condom that would be removed before entering the vagina, but even this is not foolproof for preventing vaginal infection and presents other pastoral concerns for Catholics. Considering all this, while anal penetration as part of foreplay does not appear to be *technically* forbidden by Church teaching, it is difficult to imagine any way it could be employed easily as a seamless part of foreplay leading to vaginal intercourse. From a professional perspective, I strongly discourage the practice. Nevertheless, following Augustine's dictum and in the absence of greater clarification from the Church, couples are free to prayerfully exercise prudential judgment.

allows the man to occupy the most dominant, giving posture while the woman is in the most receptive posture.

Side-by-Side Positions

Side-by-side positions can be very tender, allowing the couple to face each other and kiss intimately, or spoon together while making love. The position allows for deep emotional intimacy and gentle penetration. The position can be useful when the couple is most desirous of more cuddly intimacy or sleepy-time sex as opposed to something more energetic. In general side-by-side lovemaking is good for those times when the couple wishes to make love, but deep penetration and vigorous thrusting is undesirable (for instance, during later Phase I or pregnancy).

The position is achieved when the couple lies either facing each other or in a spooning position (man lying on his side facing the woman's back) with their legs separated enough to allow penetration. The couple can then gently thrust together.

Sitting Positions

Sitting positions can be, like the man/woman-on-top positions, very romantic and intimate, affording the couple many opportunities to kiss, caress, and gaze into each other's eyes. The position allows both the husband and wife to take nearly equal roles in determining the degree of penetration and thrusting. Some couples enjoy mutually thrusting in this position, while others prefer to simply hold each other and thrust very little for more gentle intercourse. Because it allows a great deal of control for the woman and a great deal of variation on the depth and vigorousness of penetration, sitting positions can be very good for lovemaking during Phase III and during pregnancy.

Standing Positions

Standing positions tend not be used as frequently as any of the other types of positions because they are simply not as comfortable and require some degree of dexterity. The times most couples will encounter standing positions are when they wish to make love in the shower, when the passionate couple can't quite make it to the bed, or when the couple just wants to be playful and try something different.

We have already discussed the most common standing position in which the man stands behind the woman while she bends over a bed, table, or chair (or simply leans over loosely). Other common standing positions involve the standing couple facing each other while the woman wraps one leg around the man's waist, or sits facing the man (on a table or tall stool) with the man standing in front of her. The challenge with standing positions is the height difference between the partners. The shorter partner will need to find some way to raise up high enough to achieve penetration.

SEEKING OTHER RESOURCES

This is by no means an exhaustive list, and couples should feel free to experiment with any number of creative positions that allow them to experience the fullness of their love for one another.

Additionally, couples should feel free to seek out other resources that help them discover new ways to experience the sensuality and vulnerability integral to Holy Sex. As they seek other resources, I would simply encourage couples to keep two points in mind. First, it is important to avoid inadvertently promoting pornography or casual sex. Choose sex manuals that use simple drawings and descriptions instead of photographs. Likewise, unless the models are clothed and only simulating sexual positions, avoid video presentations altogether. Although books and resources employing the explicit use of nude models can be attractively produced, they are often little more than pornography and can be very light on useful information. Even if we assumed that the couples featured in these resources are married — and that is usually difficult to believe — these materials take an intimate act that is meant to be sacred and private and make it public. Supporting such enterprises is morally highly problematic.

As long as you keep these cautions in mind, there is no need to shield yourself from all resources on sex even though they might not be completely in line with Christian teaching. Unless you personally feel that you might be led into undue temptation to engage in inappropriate actions, or unless you have access to more faithful materials that meet your needs, don't be intimidated by the fact that most books on sex will contain at least some material that is morally objectionable. Catholics can confidently make the claim that our Church contains the fullness of the truth because Catholics are open to seeking truth wherever it may be found. While Infallible Lovers should try hard to seek informational materials that contain the least amount of objectionable material, assuming that they are mature, faithful, prayerful, adults with basically well-formed consciences, there is no need to remain ignorant or in need because there are few, if any, sources of sexual information that are 100 percent pure.

Of course, no resource is more important than intimacy, respect, and good communication between you and your beloved. If you don't have these, then all the books or videos in the world won't be enough to lead you to the relationship you desire. But with such powerful resources at your disposal, you need little else to create a passionate and deeply spiritual sexual relationship that meets your needs and is uniquely your own.

Having explored various sexual positions, let's examine the sexual climax.

ACHIEVING ORGASM

Physiologically speaking, all men and women are capable of achieving orgasm, but it would be a mistake to think that orgasm is the entire point of sexual intercourse. Love and intimacy are the point of sexual intercourse. Not every sexual encounter ends in orgasm, nor does it need to.

Be that as it may, making certain that both husband and wife are as fully satisfied as they wish to be is important. Some theologians make the argument that, as a matter of justice, since sexual pleasure is a right that belongs to the state of marriage, the man has a moral duty to see that his wife is satisfied.

That does not mean that the man must keep thrusting away over and above his wife's protestations that she is perfectly content because, "Darn it all! You're not *there* yet!" Rather, it requires the husband to be attuned to the wife's needs, attentive to her desires, and aware that her arousal curve is different than his. As Karol Wojtyla wrote in *Love and Responsibility:*

> *Sexologists state that the curve of arousal in a woman is different from that in man — it rises more slowly and falls more slowly. . . . Non-observance of these teachings of sexology in the marital relationship is contrary to the good of the . . . partner . . . and to the durability and cohesion of the marriage itself. It must be taken into account that it is naturally difficult for the woman to adapt herself to the man in the sexual relationship, that there is a natural unevenness of physical and psychological rhythms, so that there is a need for harmonization, which is impossible without good will, especially on the part of the man, who must carefully observe the reactions of the woman.*

It might seem a cruel trick that God would create man and woman — who are supposed to be perfect partners for one another — to achieve climax at different times. But Wojtyla gets at the reason for this seeming contradiction in his comment about harmonization.

Infallible Lovers know that orgasm is not the point of sexual intercourse. Rather, *physical intimacy, achieved through the physical harmonization of the man and woman's arousal curve,* is the point of intercourse. To achieve this physical harmonization is to teach each other's bodies to reflect the psychological and spiritual harmonization of the partner's intimacy and friendship in their day-to-day lives. The couple's bodies then learn to be perfect helpmates to each other, just as the couple's minds and spirits have learned to be perfect helpmates during their daytime relationship.

When a man learns, and is attentive to, his wife's verbal and nonverbal pleasure cues, and he learns to synch his own arousal curve to his wife's so that they can reach the pinnacle of pleasure together, the couple has taught their *bodies* to make visible the intimate, spiritual, and psychological union that would otherwise be invisible. As Wojtyla writes,

> *...from the altruistic standpoint [that is, the point of view that requires the man to seek not primarily his own pleasure from intercourse, but rather attend to the satisfaction of his wife], it is necessary to insist that intercourse must not serve merely as a means of allowing sexual excitement to reach its climax in...the man alone, but that climax must be reached in harmony, not at the expense of one partner, but with both partners fully involved.*

(I can't resist pointing out that I have just quoted a pope preaching on the theological significance and moral desirability of simultaneous orgasm. Needless to say, this factoid is not included in the usual NACWATC Press Bulletins. Having indulged my little "toldja so" moment, we can return to the matter at hand.)

Clearly, in light of Wojtyla's statement above, to say that orgasm is not the point of Holy Sex is not the same thing as saying that climax is unimportant. Rather, Infallible Lovers know that if they teach their bodies to harmonize with each other and become more sensitive to each other's unconscious bodily cues, giving each other conscious cues when necessary, then in most cases climax — or at least mutual satisfaction — will take care of itself. Later on, in the section addressing common problems, we'll address those times when orgasm doesn't occur normally. But now let's look at how things are supposed to work in a healthy relationship.

ORGASM AND THE AROUSAL CURVE

The human arousal curve follows a similar path for both women and men, but men, without the training required of harmonization, will naturally achieve orgasm more quickly. Physiological arousal moves through the following stages first formally defined by Masters and Johnson: *Desire, Arousal, Plateau, Orgasm, and Resolution.*

253

Desire is the entry into sexual intercourse. It is purely a physiological phenomenon that can happen on its own, but Infallible Lovers often rely on their intimacy to jump-start it. When they are tired, stressed, ill, or otherwise experiencing an impairment of desire, Infallible Lovers still long for the comfort of their best friend's arms, and they trust that desire will be rekindled once they seek that comfort.

Arousal is the point when the lovers' bodies begin to respond to each other in earnest. The woman experiences increased lubrication and engorgement of her breasts, labia, and genitals. The man also experiences engorgement of the penis and erection. Men who begin to experience arousal can begin to withdraw into themselves, focusing entirely on their own pleasure rather than attending to their wives' unique pleasure cues. The man who loses himself in his own sexual experience may experience premature ejaculation shortly after this point, practically skipping right over the next stage. The man who paces himself, concentrates on slowing down his sexual responses, and adjusts position or stops for a moment when necessary (while continuing to stimulate his wife in some way) can help her arrive at the next stage with him.

Plateau is the stage of sexual excitement when the couple is within sight of climax. The penis begins to secrete pre-ejaculatory fluid which increases the woman's lubrication and allows for deeper penetration. The head of the penis becomes more engorged and the testes swell and draw up higher into the body, getting ready for ejaculation. For her part, the woman's vagina becomes even more engorged and sensitive and her clitoris begins to draw up under the clitoral hood. Her nipples become erect and areola (the dark circles around the nipples) become more sensitive to touch. For both the husband and wife, sparks are flying. The couple may wish to prolong this plateau as long as possible, enjoying the sensation that comes from standing at the edge of a cliff right before you jump off.

During Plateau, it will be especially important for the man to continue to stay focused on the woman's pleasure clues. She may become more vocal and physically active. Her vagina will become wetter and more sensitive. She may begin to arch her back to draw her pelvis closer to the man's groin. She may do many other things that are unique to her. Sometimes, Infallible Lovers may give each other small verbal cues, in a sense, checking in to see if each partner is ready to climax. If both partners are ready, the lovers will continue on. If not, the man may take a break for a moment while continuing to stimulate his wife in some other way. Remember, the goal in Holy Sex is not achieving orgasm as quickly as possible. The goal is harmonizing your bodies to reflect the intimate partnership your minds and spirits are celebrating in Holy Sex. When both are ready, they jump together from the Plateau to the next stage, orgasm.

Orgasm, the peak of the arousal curve is, for the most part, entirely beyond conscious control. Muscles now begin contracting involuntarily throughout the genitals as well as the rest of the body. The orgasm itself lasts anywhere from five to ten seconds. Immediately following climax, blood begins to return to the rest of the body. While a man will always move to the next stage, Resolution, a woman's body will often first reset to the Plateau stage, meaning that she can climax several times before achieving resolution. This is why it is the man's responsibility to learn to pace his arousal. The woman can wait for the man if she arrives at orgasm early. The man cannot.

Resolution is when the body returns to its nonaroused state. For the man, resolution involves what is known as a "refactory period" that is, the period of time nerves need to rest before they can be stimulated again. A man can go through the arousal cycle again following orgasm, but it may take some time before he can become erect again. This time increases as the man becomes older.

Exercise
LEARNING TO HARMONIZE

Because the goal of Holy Sex is harmonization of the body's responses so that even their bodies can reflect the intimate partnership the couple shares all day, take a moment to reflect on each other's pleasure cues that accompany each stage. Respond to the following questions and discuss them with your spouse to help you and your mate become more in synch with each other.

1. Think about those times when each of you begins to feel sexually *desirous* of your mate. How do you begin acting toward your partner? What behaviors do you display? Are there certain things you say? How about body language?

2. Think about those times when each of you begins to feel *actively aroused* by your mate. How do you begin acting toward your partner? What behaviors do you display? Are there certain things you say? Consider your body language. Do your bodies begin changing in some noticeable way?

Before considering the next stage, Plateau, think about ways that you help pace yourselves so that you can stay in synch with each other. If you struggle with this, what are some things you would like the husband to do to pause his own ascent up the arousal curve (e.g., withdraw for a moment, pause in thrusting, focus on slowing breathing) while he continues to stimulate the wife (e.g., genitally, orally, or manually), allowing her to "catch up"?

3. Think about those times when each of you reach Plateau, the point where climax is in sight, but still consciously preventable. How do you begin acting toward your partner? What behaviors do you display? Are there certain things you say? How about body language? Are there noticeable changes in your bodies?

Before considering the next stage, Orgasm, consider ways that you help pace yourselves so that you can stay in synch with each other.

4. Think about the times when you achieve the next stage, Orgasm, with your spouse. Reflect on times that have been especially intense and satisfying. Is there anything you like your spouse to do for you while you are climaxing? Is there anything your partner could do to intensify the experience of your orgasm?

5. After you have achieved orgasm, during the Resolution Stage what makes you feel closest to your mate? If there are several things, describe when — generally speaking — you most prefer the things you listed.

Note: For additional tips on harmonization of the sexual response cycle, please review the section on premature ejaculation (pp. 291 below).

BECOMING MORE SEXUALLY PRESENT

In the previous exercise, you identified the different ways that you could harmonize your experience of arousal during intercourse. A big part of being able to achieve this goal is attending to what your partner needs from you in the moment more than you are attending to your own pleasure. This is not to say that you should not be concerned with your own pleasure, but there is a paradox. The more focused the partners are on their own pleasure during sex, the less intimate and pleasurable sex becomes.

The Catholic solution to this problem is something called "mutual self-donation." Mutual self-donation is a way to make sure that both the husband and the wife get all of their needs met without either one having to be selfish about it. It is a kind of heroic generosity that views everything we have (including our bodies) as a gift God gives to us, but asks us to hold in trust for others so that we can use those gifts to work for their good. My talents, my treasure, even my body, are not entirely mine to do with completely as I please. More accurately, rather than the owner, I am the steward of these things. While I may use them in a way that is beneficial to me, I must do so in a manner that is primarily beneficial to others. This applies to every aspect of life of course, but let's take a moment to spell out how this works when applied to the sexual relationship.

Lesser lovers are primarily concerned with protecting themselves. Even in the absence of conflicts over moral absolutes, they bristle at being asked to leave their comfort zone. They approach each other with an attitude that says, "I'm here to see to my satisfaction or comfort." They try to make sure their mate gets something out of the deal, but they are mainly concerned with getting their own needs met.

By contrast, Infallible Lovers who practice mutual self-donation say, "Everything I have and everything I am is yours." They work hard to learn what their mate needs and hold themselves accountable for doing these things, often without being asked, and certainly without having to be asked twice (the Daily Marital Checkup, p. 213, is a great way to maintain this accountability). When a couple practices mutual self-donation, they are happy to tell each other what they need as often as necessary, but then they focus primarily on meeting the other's needs, trusting that their own needs will be met in turn. This way, each lover gets all of his or her needs met without having to be selfish or self-protective.

I talk to many couples in my counseling practice who think this is a lovely ideal that simply cannot be achieved. And then, after much wrangling, I get them to do it, and they are shocked at how happy they can make each other. Mutual self-donation takes work. It takes trust. It takes commitment. It takes guts. But then, Infallible Loving is not for those who are lazy, untrustworthy, uncommitted, or gutless.

If you are man or woman enough to take on the challenge of mutual self-donation — and reap the rewards from the risk — complete the following exercise.

SEXUAL LOVELIST

Earlier, you completed a Lovelist exercise that consisted of listing twenty-five things that make you feel loved in your day-to-day relationship (see p. 214). Now we will apply this same exercise to your sexual relationship.

The first step in self-donation is being able to express to your mate the ways that he or she can please you. After all, your mate cannot know how best to make a gift out of himself or herself unless you make your needs and desires known. Take a moment to reflect on the times when you feel closest during lovemaking and the things your mate does — or could do — that would be most meaningful during lovemaking. There are only two rules to consider in making your list. First, you may not list any activity that you know to be opposed to the One Rule. Second, be positive and specific. Ask for the things that you *do* want, not the things you wish your mate would stop doing. This exercise is not intended to be a complaint list. It is an invitation to love each other better.

List at least twenty-five ways your mate can please you most during fore-play and lovemaking. When your lists are completed exchange lists with your mate. Remember, assuming that your mate has not listed anything that violates the One Rule, the heroic generosity that lies at the heart of self-donation requires you to at least be willing charitably to consider fulfilling all the items on your mate's lovelist. In the event you have questions or concerns about something your mate is asking for, use the steps for negotiating sexual differences identified in our previous discussion on the Four Pleasure Principles (pp. 192ff.).

Each time you make love, try to make sure that you do at least one of the things on your mate's list that comes easily to you *and* one thing that represents a challenge to your comfort zone. Be sure to pray about these items, and use your Daily Marital Checkups (p. 213) to discuss any ongoing concerns about the continuity between your day-to-day relationship and your sexual relationship.

AFTERGLOW

After a couple makes love, they experience an increase in hormones like oxytocin that make them feel mellower and closer to each other. Oxytocin also helps people deal more calmly with petty irritations that come up in relationships. As we have discussed previously, that is why so many couples who rarely, if ever, communicate, relate, or pray together rely so heavily upon sex to hold them together.

But when Infallible Lovers celebrate Holy Sex, they place lovemaking in the context of a wider relationship founded upon all the virtues that enable them to live life as a gift. In this context, God gives couples the ability to harmonize their bodies in such a way that the bonding hormones they produce during the celebration of Holy Sex help them find the strength to become even more perfect in love. We discussed this dynamic at length when we considered the Fourth Power of Holy Sex, the power to unite, but it bears repeating here now that we have walked through the process by which this unity is achieved.

Secular readers will be interested to know that the intimate cyclical relationship between arousal and emotional intimacy, which I just described as the traditional view of Holy Sex, is now considered to be cutting edge information in the field of modern sexology. The journals *Sexual and Relationship Therapy* and the *Journal of Sex and Marital Therapy* have both published research on what is known as the Basson Sexual Response Cycle (BSRC). This is a new model of secular sex therapy that eschews sexology's previous assumptions about sex driven by physical desire alone. Rather, researcher Rosemary Basson describes the sexual relationship as a continuum between intimacy and arousal and notes that, in long-term relationships especially, it is intimacy that activates the process of desire, which then leads to a closer physical connection that, in turn, promotes greater intimacy. Pretty much what Catholics have been saying all along and what Infallible Lovers have known since the beginning of time. It's good to have the research to confirm it, but once again, the modern scientist ascends the mountain of inquiry to find that someone else has beaten him to it and built a cathedral while waiting.

Work, Work, Work

Some people might be led to ask, "Why is all this so much work?" Speaking about the Theology of the Body, Pope John Paul II pointed out that before the Fall, our first parents lived in original unity — experiencing a total harmonization within themselves and with each other. The *work* contemporary men and women must do to synchronize their bodies, minds, and spirits is the result of dis-integration of both the human person and the relationship between man and woman caused by original sin. But God, in his mercy, gives us the sacrament of marriage to help men and women reestablish as much of that original unity as we can on this side of heaven. When Infallible Lovers teach their bodies to make visible the invisible unity they experience in their daily life, and then use the physiological boost their bodies give them to challenge each other to grow more completely in perfection and love, they activate the spiritual, psychological, relational, and physiological machinery by which husbands and wives can become much more than Infallible Lovers: *they can become saints.*

That is why the Church is so "hung up" about sex.

And that is why you should be, too.

The path to becoming Infallible Lovers is, as St. Thérèse of Lisieux might put it, the "little way" toward the sanctification of the married couple and the means by which the sacrament of marriage transforms men and women into saints. Holy Sex involves much more than recreation. It truly does involve the re-creation of the wedding day in which man and woman promised one another in the sight of God and his Church to help each other become everything God created them to be in this life — body, mind, and spirit — and prepare each other to attend the heavenly wedding feast with their Divine Lover in the next.

PART FOUR

Overcoming
Common Problems

Now that you have seen how Holy Sex works, the next several chapters will offer technical support for those couples who are struggling to make it work for them.

14   IS THERE SEX AFTER KIDS?

Whoever welcomes a little child welcomes me.

— Matthew 18:5

I hear it all the time: "Children change everything." There's a popular notion that marriage can be divided into two epochs, B.C. ("Before Children") and A.D. ("After Diapers"). The B.C. marriage is allegedly a time of wanton romance and joy: candlelight dinners, violins, dancing till dawn, and all the things that "true love" entails. The A.D. marriage is what happens when people settle down and get responsible, boring, and old. According to popular culture, the A.D. marriage is the beginning of the end of the passion. This is the time when the couple starts paying exclusive attention to raising the kids (and paying for them) and becomes too busy, too tired, and too distracted for anything like romance. It doesn't have to be that way.

Many couples actually have stronger marital friendships because they have children together. Many couples actually grow in love with each other because they have added children to the family. What gives these couples the strength to buck the conventional wisdom? It would seem that it is largely up to the husbands.

Too often, husbands leave romance up to the wife. In many marriages, it is the wife who plans date night, makes the plans for the romantic dinner or that special event, and makes sure they take time for conversation and prayer. By contrast, the husband is the passive beneficiary of his wife's loving effort. Then along comes baby, and all of a sudden, the woman is preoccupied with a little person who can't take care of himself—and no, I don't mean her husband. In the presence of this reality, the husband may respond in one of two ways—with jealousy or with love. If the husband chooses jealousy over love, he will respond to the baby as a threat. The more involved the mother is with their child, the more he may act as if he feels himself to be an outsider. He may intentionally withdraw from child-care as a way to protest her "betrayal." He may begin insisting that she make time for dates or sex before it is even physically possible or emotionally prudent. If she is anything but wildly enthusiastic about his proposals, he may act like a pouting child who has been disciplined unjustly. If this pattern keeps up, the wife comes to see her husband as "another child" whom she has to "take care of." She learns to view romance, and especially sex, as "one more chore." Barring a dramatic change, these marriages can devolve more and more into a brother-sister relationship that is tinged by resentment as neither the wife nor the husband is getting their own needs for intimacy and support met.

The second option is for the husband to take advantage of the opportunity for love that has been presented to him with the birth of this child. In this scenario, the husband sees it as his responsibility to take as good care of the wife and marriage as she is taking care of their child. He compliments her on her mothering and actively looks for ways to support and encourage her in the tiring job of tending to the baby. He reminds her that she's beautiful, but not in a way that implies that her beauty makes her an object to him. He reminds her that, in addition to being a mother, she is a woman with a mind and heart and soul, but he is careful to do this in a way that does not give the impression that he is taking care of her so that he can get something out of her. In other words, the parenting role calls both husband and wife to different forms of a very selfless kind of loving. If the husband responds to the wife in this manner, the wife will come to see her relationship with her husband as a safe haven, a retreat, the one place she can go to rest and feel cared for and recuperate from her long day of caring for another. As she relaxes in her husband's arms at the end of a long day, her romantic response to him will emerge as a logical response to his having loved her first, and loved her well.

I have found that it is in this kind of environment — one in which husband and wife truly see themselves as partners in the raising and caring of the children — that a truly loving openness to life will grow. This is also why it is so common for NFP couples to want to keep having children after they have the societal norm of two or three kids.

There are those who think the dynamic I describe is too "pie-in-the-sky," but research supports that it is possible to achieve greater intimacy after baby (or babies). Gottman's study, *Bringing Baby Home,* found that when husbands were as emotionally clued in to the marital relationship as their wives and, as I described in the second option above, actively engaged in infant care, those couples actually became more intimate as their family size increased. Why? Because these couples see the parenting role as one more thing that draws them together, and the wife comes to be grateful to the husband for his loving, selfless attention to her, which then gives her the emotional peace and security she needs to be the point person for a great deal of the direct care of the baby.

In two-career families, the husband's active role is even more critical. In her book *Second Shift* sociologist Arlie Hochschild notes that despite society's talk about equality of roles, most women who work outside the home are still responsible for the lion's share of domestic chores and child-rearing. In this dynamic, the marriage and the sexual relationship suffer horribly as the wife comes to see taking care of her husband the chore that is last on the list. By contrast, research shows that in two-career marriages in which the husband is an active partner in childrearing and chores, the marital intimacy also increases because of, rather than in spite of, children.

Of course, the idea that marital intimacy should increase with the advent of children completely gels with Catholic teaching. As you've read throughout this book, the family images the Trinity who — beginning as a powerful and intimate community of love — creates new life, brings that creation back into itself, and then is inspired (in a sense) by the now-greater community of love to create more life. And so on, and so on. The family images the Trinity in that it too is, ideally, an ever-expanding example of love which gives life, brings that life back into itself, and is inspired by the intimacy experienced within that community to create more life, and so on, and so on.

Science and the Church agree. When husbands take their godly place as servant-leaders in their home, acting like men who can love and care for their wives and be intimate partners to their wives, instead of becoming children who must be placated and pacified by wifely attention, marriages become stronger as the family increases.

15 WHEN NFP IS TOO HARD

A tree is shown by its fruits, and in the same way, those who profess to belong to Christ will be seen by what they do. For what is needed is not mere present profession, but perseverance to the end in the power of faith.

— St. Ignatius of Antioch

Marcia called my radio program with a question about NFP. "It just doesn't work for us."

I smelled a rat, but I played along. "Hmm. Tell me a little bit more about what you mean by that."

"Well, we have five kids with it."

"Oh," I answered, still suspicious but trying hard to be nice. "You mean all five children were a complete surprise?"

"Well, um, no," she replied. "But y'know, my husband has a really strong, um, libido. And so we can't do NFP."

Okay. Let's stop here. There are about a hundred directions we could go with this, but I want to highlight one part of this couple's experience because it is something I hear a great deal about from my clients and callers. Specifically, I am referring to the objection that NFP doesn't work because some men — and women — find it "too frustrating." It would be easy to belittle such comments, but it would be wrong to do so. The struggle with our fallen selves is a serious matter, and there is real pain involved. Sexual frustration can be the source of great tension in a marriage, and unless a couple understands it and knows what to do with it, the person's mental health and marriage will suffer.

As I indicated above, this is a big question, and there are more dimensions to this problem than we can adequately deal with in the space I have here. To make things more manageable, let's focus this discussion on the relationship between sexual frustration and NFP. In *Love and Responsibility* as well as his reflections on the Theology of the Body, John Paul II teaches that sexual attraction serves both as a reminder that we were not created to be alone and as a call to remember that we are always to work for the good of the other. In other words, as long as our sexual energy and urges inspire us to draw closer to our mate *and* keep our mate's best interest in mind simultaneously, then those urges are good and godly. By contrast, if our urges cause us to be primarily concerned with getting what I "need" from my spouse no matter what, then that urge is disordered, fallen, and ungodly. Left unchecked, that urge can ultimately destroy my marriage and my soul.

As I am fond of reminding people, NFP is not, in my view, primarily a means of spacing children. It is, in my view, primarily a spiritual exercise that allows couples to accomplish three ends: (1) to facilitate the communication and prayer life of the couple, (2) to help the couple prayerfully discern their family size and, on an ongoing basis, continue to both balance and expand all the virtues associated with the unity and procreativity inherent in marriage, and (3) to help the couple achieve holiness, freedom, and true love through self-mastery and self-control.

It is point (3) that I am most concerned with here. All of us are broken. All of us struggle with the desire to use another for our own selfish ends. For some, that struggle against selfishness is more difficult than for others, but it's in all of us, and overcoming it is hard and sometimes painful. The spiritual beauty of NFP is that it highlights that struggle and challenges us to overcome our tendencies toward selfishness in ways we might not otherwise be challenged. When someone says that NFP "doesn't work" for them because they get too sexually frustrated, I have to respond that, in fact, NFP was *made* for them. Why? Because any sexual urge that — if unsatisfied — threatens to blot out all the other good things about the marriage is a disordered urge that will destroy the person, the couple, or both. Such an urge must be tamed.

Is this unrealistic? No. As you discovered earlier in this book, the sexual drive is part of the neuroendocrine system, the same primitive brain system responsible for urges like hunger and anger. What person in his right mind would argue that intense urges to rage at people indiscriminately or eat uncontrollably should be encouraged? No one. In fact, we praise people who have mastered these urges for being in some ways more human than those who have not mastered them. I don't mean they have *repressed* these urges, mind you, but rather that they have developed the capacity to consciously choose when to use them and when not to. Likewise, people who have mastered these urges — who are capable of eating or stopping *as they choose* or being angry or not *as they choose* — can be said to be *more free* than people who must eat any time the urge strikes or must rage any time their anger is pricked.

And here is the irony. Although society makes a distinction between the sex drive and the anger and hunger drives, the brain does not. Society praises the unfettered sex drive, while practically criminalizing people who are overweight. But the same region of the brain is responsible for all three urges. Gaining mastery over our sex drive — that is, being able to consciously choose to use it only when it is ordered toward the good of the other person — makes us *more human* and *more free* than the person who must give in to every impulse for sex "or else." Having to wrestle with this fallen nature is hard. The process is painful but it is *sanctifying,* and that struggle is a necessary part of the daily life of anyone who takes his or her mental and spiritual health seriously.

We need to recognize that any frustration we feel in the process of doing NFP is a sign that NFP *is working.* When we feel those pains, we must learn to recognize them as the growing pains that accompany both our advancing spiritual maturity and our increasing capacity for true love (i.e., the ability to work for the good of the other even when doing so makes us uncomfortable). In those times when the growing pains — the disordered sexual frustration — hurt the most, we must recognize that we are not feeling a sexual urge that must be satisfied, but feeling a selfish urge that must be contained and transformed. In response, we must draw closer to our mate, in conversation, prayer, work, and nonsexual affection, as a way of reclaiming the freedom that our fallenness has taken from us. Is it always easy? Absolutely not, and anyone who says otherwise is telling you a tale. But it is worth it, because with the struggle comes an increased capacity to become the lover, the person, and the child of God each of us is being called to be.

DEALING WITH FRUSTRATION

All of this leads to the obvious question, "How can a couple effectively deal with the frustration they may experience during the phases when they choose to abstain from lovemaking?" Obviously, some couples do better than others. What are the differences that help some couples handle periodic abstinence better than others?

1. Pray Together

To do NFP well, and especially to receive the grace and develop the strength to handle periodic abstinence well, a couple must be praying together constantly. I never stop being amazed at how many couples — even NFP-practicing couples who have been taught about the importance of prayer — simply do not pray *together.* Almost as bad, I have met too many couples who pray in a very perfunctory manner that does not actually bring their real life, joys, and pains before the Lord. If you are not praying with your spouse, especially about your sexual life together, then it will be too easy to forget that the main reason you are abstaining in a given month is not because you don't want more children right now (this is supposed to have very little to do with your will), but because God has asked you to take some time off from your sexual relationship to grow in particular virtues as a couple, as a family, or as a person. Only through constant prayer and seeking God's will for both your own life and your life as a couple will you be able to discern the specific reasons God is asking you to abstain for a specific period of time. The frustration of periodic abstinence is always easier to bear when you can see the fruit God will bring out of it, and when you can cry to him — together — when it seems too hard.

271

2. Talk Openly, Honestly, and without Blaming

Couples who handle periodic abstinence better than others make the time to talk regularly (at least several times a week) with each other, not just about what things need to be accomplished and what is going on in their children's lives, but also about their emotional and spiritual health and where they think God is leading them as individuals and as a couple. They also talk openly, without blaming the other or becoming defensive, about their personal struggles with sexual frustration and the pain that is a natural part of growing into the people God is calling them to be. These latter conversations take the form of personal statements such as, "I know God has asked us to take this time off, but sometimes it hurts so much when I just want to be with you." And *not* statements like, "You're always saying 'no' to me. Why can't you just loosen up!" Or, "Why do you have to be so legalistic about this? Can't we just use a condom this time?"

3. Be Affectionate

Couples who do poorly handling the frustration of periodic abstinence tend almost completely to avoid sharing any kinds of affection with each other unless it's going to lead to sex. These couples will say things like "I can't hug you in Phase II, because if I do, I get too crazy." Or, as one acquaintance of mine put it, "I can work late for the next couple of nights because we're in Phase II, so it's not like we can do anything anyway." Such avoidance of real, nonsexual intimacy points directly to a truly immature view of sexuality that is more about self-indulgence than self-giving.

By contrast, couples who handle the frustration of periodic abstinence well are always as affectionate as they can be throughout all the phases of their cycle. These couples know that hugs, kisses, cuddling, and even "making out" don't have to end in sex, and in fact it can be a real aphrodisiac when they don't. As I mentioned in an earlier chapter, when a couple enters sex therapy (even secular sex therapy, with all its baggage), one of the first things the therapist will do is tell the couple to stop having sex for a while so that they can work on increasing the nonsexual affection that creates the safe, loving, and nurturing environment necessary for a vital sexual relationship to flourish. This exercise is called sensate focus. But it's really just a clinical manifestation of the SPICE habits we discussed in our examination of the benefits of NFP (pp. 172ff.). Couples who handle periodic abstinence better than others follow the counterintuitive rule that the more affectionate they are (despite having been led by God to abstain for a time), the easier the abstinence will be.

4. Make Sex Part of the Larger Whole

The simple fact is that if you experience NFP as "ruining your marriage," you have bigger problems than NFP. In fact, as you might guess from reading this far, I would argue that your problems with NFP are simply symbolic of your struggles to communicate effectively, pray together effectively, or share (nonsexual) intimacy. Although it will always be a challenge to some degree or another, the couple who successfully negotiates the challenges of periodic abstinence is the couple that clearly recognizes sex as the tip of the larger iceberg representing their daily communication and spiritual and intimate life. Such couples don't think of their sexual relationship as a thing that can or should stand on its own. They genuinely see sex as an expression of the deep prayer life, solid communication, common intimacy, and uncommon partnership that they celebrate in their daily lives together — and because of this, they don't take these elements for granted. Because they are already excellent partners in these areas, being partners in the pursuit of continence, self-control, and true love comes much more naturally.

It's always easier to kill the messenger than to heed the message. If NFP is challenging you and your marriage, *good*. It's doing what it's supposed to do. Have courage and do the work it is calling you to do, and know that as a reward for your struggle, you'll become a healthier, more godly person, and have a more intimate and godly marriage.

UNEQUALLY YOKED — WHEN YOU CAN'T AGREE ON NFP

Here's another way that NFP can be "hard on a marriage": when one spouse sees the wisdom of using it, but the other spouse is vehemently opposed. The following email I received from a woman who read my book *Beyond the Birds and the Bees* is a good example of this problem.

> *I've gotten more serious about my faith in the last year or so. I've done a lot of reading, and God's really opened my eyes about how Natural Family Planning is the way to go. The problem is my husband is absolutely, completely, 100 percent against it. I don't know what to do. I don't think the time is right for more children, but I can't bring myself to contracept. But my husband says he'd rather never have sex again than trust NFP. What do I do?*

My wife and I get calls exactly like this on our radio program almost every day. And a surprising number of husbands call us to say that it is the wife who is the reluctant partner. But whoever plays the role of the hold-out in your home, the question is the same: How do you maintain your integrity while respecting that your spouse is at a different stage of his or her faith journey?

This is a sticky question, and since there are so many variations on the theme, here are five general guidelines to help you figure out the best way through this problem in your marriage.

1. Don't Go It Alone

My first piece of advice for you is don't try to do this by yourself. There are so many different objections spouses can offer, and so many different responses you should or should not make based upon your unique circumstances, that it's essential to enlist good pastoral guidance. I would strongly encourage you to talk on a regular basis with your pastor, your teaching couple, the good people at the Couple-to-Couple League (*www.ccli.org*), or a pastoral counselor familiar with the unique concerns of NFP couples.

The questions and issues that emerge are serious, and the way you respond to the challenges you face will affect the tone of your marriage for years to come. Get faithful support and counsel.

So how do you know how serious your situation is? Think of it this way. While some degree of questioning is perfectly natural when a spouse suddenly announces, "Guess what, Honey? I've signed us up for an NFP class!" if your spouse digs in and fights you tooth and nail, this is really not an NFP problem so much as a marriage problem touching on deep issues of respect, communication, and spirituality. Because these are such hot button issues, it's important to get competent counsel to know how to respond charitably and sanely. Don't be too proud to ask for help early in this process.

2. Know the Parameters

The Congregation for the Doctrine of the Faith published a document called the *Vademecum for Confessors Concerning Some Aspects of the Morality of Conjugal Life*. I'll summarize the high points.

First, it's best when both spouses agree to use only licit ways to regulate conception (NFP). If one spouse is being stubborn about this, it would be preferable for the faithful spouse to abstain from sexual relations altogether. If this isn't possible, then for "grave reasons," the faithful spouse may engage in sexual relations with the contracepting spouse *but only* if three conditions are met.

1. The faithful spouse is not the one using any form of artificial birth control.

2. There must be grave, morally clear reasons that there is no other prudent option available to the faithful spouse. Remember, it's your job to be able to justify these reasons before the Lord. Make sure you can.

3. The faithful spouse must commit to an ongoing effort to change the heart of the reluctant spouse and be actively working to get their marriage in order with God's plan for their sexual relationship over time.

There is one other consideration. The above three conditions do not apply to situations where the Pill or other chemical birth control is used, because these methods can cause abortion. The *Vademecum* insists on "careful evaluation" by a competent spiritual authority (i.e., a faithful pastor) whenever chemical abortifacients are being used. Generally, though, you most likely may not engage in sexual relations if there is a possibility of any fertilized egg being aborted (prevented from implantation by artificial hormonal contraception).

So, assuming you are not using abortifacients (like the Pill or other hormonal contraceptives), the Church gives you a little room in which to work.

Nevertheless, I almost always encourage my clients in this situation to insist on abstaining from sexual relations except in infertile times. The reason I advise this is that when a spouse insists on using artificial contraception over your objections, that spouse is saying that he or she has the right to do whatever he or she wants with his or her body *and* yours. No spouse has that right. This is a serious spiritual and psychological offence against your personhood. The Church teaches that the only right husbands and wives have over each other is the right to work for each other's good. When your spouse insists on contracepting, your spouse is offending your dignity and his or her own. Even though it will be difficult, the only truly loving, godly thing to do is to say, "No. I love you too much to allow you to do this to yourself and to me." Sometime, love must be tough. This is one of those times.

3. Be Assertive

Every time I'm asked to address this question, I ask the person, "Have you and your spouse signed up for an NFP course?" Over and over again, the answer is, "No. He (she) says that he won't go."

Here is my advice. Don't ask permission. Sign up for the course, and tell your spouse when it is. Don't give your spouse a chance to say no. You are working for the good of your marriage and for the good of your mate's soul. Don't be afraid to push a little. Of course, if they lock themselves in the bathroom and barricade the door the day of your class, I'm not suggesting that you make them go (although if your mate is really that immature, you really do need to be in marital counseling as of yesterday). But make it clear that short of such histrionics, your mate is expected to be there. If you want to be taken seriously, you must let your mate know that you are deadly serious about this.

4. Do This in Love

Acting from love is key. At the same time that you're being Captain Assertive, it is your obligation to turn up the (nonsexual) love in your marriage. Exponentially.

Think of those thousand or so (nonsexual) things your spouse has asked you to do for him or her, but you have been dragging your feet. Start doing them today. Furthermore, promise yourself and God right now that you're going to commit to doing these things every day for the rest of your life whether or not your spouse ever changes.

Why?

Two reasons. First, if you're inviting your mate to express the kind of generosity that NFP requires without being willing to model that same generosity in every area of your marriage, then you're going to look like you're running for hypocrite of the year. You have no credibility. Zero. Too many spouses sit in their own marital sloth complaining about their stubborn mate, when they themselves aren't lifting a finger to love as God calls them to love. Don't let this be you, because this is the sin of spiritual pride, and pride is the deadliest of the deadly sins.

Second, you need to do this because your spouse needs to understand that your desire to do NFP is not coming from your recent discovery of some obscure (and bizarre) set of rules invented by celibate men on some far-off planet. Your spouse must understand — on an experiential level — that your desire to use NFP is motivated by your sincere desire to love him (or her) even better than you already do. To establish this context, you must be loving in every way you can even while insisting on NFP. Mind you, I'm not suggesting that you try to "buy" or manipulate your spouse's agreement. Rather, I am asserting that the only godly way to motivate a conversion to the truth is through love. You can win over their heart through your genuinely loving example. You may not browbeat your mate into NFP submission and expect to get any marital or spiritual "points" for this kind of behavior. You might as well pat yourself on the back for baptizing your neighbors at gunpoint. Catholic moral teaching tells us that it's never acceptable to attempt to accomplish a good goal (even a goal as good as NFP compliance) using evil means.

Now do you see why I want you to seek counsel?

5. PRAY PRAY PRAY PRAY PRAY

Did I mention that you should be giving this problem to God every single day? I'm constantly amazed by the people who offer stunned silence when I ask them, "So are you praying about this?"

Make no mistake. The acceptance of NFP in marriage is about nothing if not conversion. It is the Holy Spirit, not you, who effects conversion. If you ain't prayin', then conversion probably ain't happ'nin'.

The bottom line is that you *can* do this. In fact, I help couples make this transition every day. And if they can do it, so can you.

Just remember, the generosity required by this transition doesn't come naturally or easily. Even so, if by God's grace and your commitment to cooperating with that grace you're able to make this shift in your marriage, then you will not be sorry. Indeed, you'll be happier than ever because you won't just be slavishly "doing NFP." You'll be living in the generous, intimate partnership to which NFP calls you.

16 YOU'VE LOST THAT LOVING FEELING

Like attraction, desire is of the essence of love. . . . Desire too belongs to the very essence of the love which springs up between a man and woman.
— Karol Wojtyla, *Love and Responsibility*

M aria, forty-two, has been married to Chuck for twenty years. "I just don't have the same drive I used to when I was younger. Between the children, and work, and life, I just don't feel 'it' so much anymore. Chuck gets mad at me when I tell him I'm not interested, but what does he want? For me to lie? I just don't feel aroused like I used to. I love him and all. But we're just not kids anymore. I wish he could just understand. I guess that's just the way men are."

◆ ◆ ◆

Helena, forty-three, is married to George and has been for twenty-two years. She's worried there's something wrong with her husband. "He just couldn't care less about sex. Nothing happens unless I practically throw myself at him. It didn't use to be like this. I try to talk to him, but he just won't talk about it. I've asked him to see a doctor — I've heard that some men lose testosterone when they hit middle-age — but he'll never go. When I try to cuddle up at night, he just says, 'I'm tired' and rolls over. I go between thinking that there's something wrong, to thinking there's someone else, to worrying that he's using pornography or something. This just isn't normal! Guys are supposed to want sex all the time. Right?"

According to research, low sexual desire (Hypoactive Sexual Desire Disorder — HSDD) affects up to 30 percent of women and up to 15 percent of men. In the last several years, the treatment of sexual issues related to low desire has become something of a publishing cottage industry.

In this chapter, we'll briefly examine the common causes of HSDD and possible treatment options.

MEDICAL AND PHARMACOLOGICAL CONCERNS

For women, a decrease in desire can be related to the hormonal shifts following birth, lactation, perimenopause, menopause, and hysterectomy. Hypothyroidism (low thyroid) and diabetes may also negatively affect desire. According to research published in the journal *Psychoneuro-endocrinology*, oral contraceptives have a strong negative affect on sexual desire. Studies report that oral contraceptives are responsible for up to 13 percent of cases of HSDD in women, despite advertising that implies that hormonal contraceptives give her greater sexual freedom since they can limit the number of periods a woman has. It is ironic, then, that with this increased "freedom" can come the lack of desire to enjoy the freedom. This is one more reason why NFP is a remarkably better option for women's health and relational well-being.

Since hormone replacement therapy has been discredited, there are few pharmacological options for women who experience HSDD as the result of estrogen depletion encountered during perimenopause and menopause. There are, however, nutritional options that can yield a great benefit. The book *Fertility, Cycles, and Nutrition* by Marylin Shannon is an excellent resource for women who would like to pursue natural options of treating this and many other sexual issues.

Scientists are still searching for the medical basis of HSDD in men. According to the *British Journal of Urology International*, previous thinking that HSDD was related to low testosterone levels has been largely discounted, since even men who have comparatively low levels of the hormone have more than enough for healthy sexual function. Previous studies have shown that when men are given mega-doses of testosterone, they experience a heightened state of arousal, but this does not translate to a greater amount of sexual activity or a greater number of erections. This leads researchers to believe that emotional and relationship issues figure prominently in the presence of HSDD for both women and men.

One other medical factor affecting desire for both men and women is antidepressant use, which is well-known to have negative sexual side effects.

Although the best research available points to psychological and relational causes for HSDD, it's always good to check with your physician before ruling out medical factors.

PSYCHOLOGICAL AND RELATIONSHIP FACTORS

Regardless of the use of antidepressants, clinical depression itself can strongly decrease sexual desire. If a person experiences low sexual desire in addition to difficulties enjoying other previously enjoyable activities, the tendency to avoid social situations, difficulties concentrating or motivating oneself, increased irritability, or significant changes in eating or sleep patterns, it would be wise to seek an evaluation for the possibility of depression.

We've already discussed more common psychological and relational factors affecting sexual desire. If you think that arousal rather than intimacy should drive sexual desire, you're setting yourself up for HSDD. If you struggle with shame about the body or discomfort with sexuality, you'll experience impaired desire. If a couple neglects their emotional, spiritual, and psychological intimacy or is experiencing high levels of conflict, they too are at high risk for HSDD. Likewise, if the couple thinks of sex as simply "one more nice thing to do at the end of the day" instead of "the way we celebrate the intimacy we experience all day long," they are at high risk for HSDD.

Infallible Lovers who are knowledgeable about Holy Sex simply don't experience HSDD with the same frequency that lesser lovers do. If you've ruled out the significant medical and clinical factors affecting HSDD and you're still experiencing low desire, go back through the sections of this book dealing with social intercourse. If you'd like additional support exploring the psychological and relational factors that may be decreasing your desire, contact the Pastoral Solutions Institute to see how faithful, competent counseling may assist you in achieving the passion God wills for your marriage.

17 COMMON SEXUAL PROBLEMS FOR WOMEN

It is necessary to insist that intercourse must not serve as a means of allowing climax in . . . the man alone, but that climax must be reached in harmony, not at the expense of one partner, but with both partners fully involved. — Karol Wojtyla, *Love and Responsibility*

Painful intercourse and difficulties achieving orgasm are two of the most common problems associated with women's enjoyment of sex. This chapter considers some of the causes of these problems, as well as simple strategies for resolving them.

PAINFUL INTERCOURSE

Women experience painful intercourse in many different ways. It can be felt as searing pain, or burning sensations, or intense cramping during intercourse. It can be felt either externally, in the vulva, or deep inside the vagina or abdomen.

The most frequent cause of painful intercourse is a lack of sufficient lubrication. This could be the result of an insufficient amount of foreplay, unhealthy thoughts and feelings about sex, relationship problems, medication reactions, the changes in hormone levels during perimenopause or menopause, or some combination of the above. When painful intercourse is the result of a lack of lubrication, you may correct this problem by taking more time with foreplay, using strategies described in our previous discussion of foreplay to increase the variety of stimulation during the period leading up to intercourse, and the use of over-the-counter personal lubricants.

Other causes of painful intercourse can include infections or rashes, problems with the actual structure of the vagina (including episiotomy scarring), allergies to chemical contraception (spermicides) or over-the-counter personal lubricants, sexually transmitted diseases, the thinning and stretching of the vaginal wall caused by low estrogen levels, or past sexual trauma.

Any time a woman consistently experiences painful intercourse, she should seek an evaluation by her gynecologist. Because there are so many possible causes, it's important to get a proper evaluation by a competent physician so that an appropriate course of treatment can be determined.

PROBLEMS WITH ORGASM

"My husband and I have been married for five years, and we have one child. The problem is that I've never had a climax in all the years of our marriage. My husband tries hard to please me, but nothing seems to make a difference. It's gotten to the point where I am almost repulsed by sex. I dread our time together, and sometimes I wish we never had to do it again. I don't understand what's wrong with me. What can I do?"

Many women do not have an orgasm every time they have sex, and in most cases this is not a problem. A woman can achieve at least some measure of satisfaction even if she does not climax. According to a study in the journal *Sexualities, Evolution and Gender,* some women who are generally satisfied with their sexual relationship feel that the absence of an orgasm in a particular instance of lovemaking is not a significant concern.

Surveys consistently show that about 10 percent of women have never experienced orgasm, and up to 40 percent of women experience orgasm infrequently and are dissatisfied as a result. Female Orgasmic Disorder, or anorgasmia, are the names of the condition that results when the woman's inability to achieve orgasm — either for a period of time or for the duration of her marriage — becomes problematic for the woman's psychological or relational well-being.

The good news is that this is a highly treatable problem, though it often requires professional assistance to resolve. Women who struggle with anorgasmia should feel confident in seeking the help they may need, for even Pope John Paul II encouraged those who struggle with the gift of sexuality to seek professional assistance, provided that the advice given is respectful of Catholic sexual ethics (see *Love and Responsibility*).

If you experience problems related to the absence of orgasms, the first thing you need to do is to make an appointment with your gynecologist to see if there is any physical obstacle to intimacy. While this is not usually the cause, it's important to rule out medical causes before pursuing the psychological treatments available. Assuming, however, that you're in good health, problems achieving climax tend to stem from one of (or some combination of) these five problem areas.

Problems with Technique

Most incidents of Female Orgasmic Disorder are caused by psychological issues or relationship problems, but sometimes anorgasmia can simply be the result of a problem with technique. As a first order of treatment, couples should use the harmonization exercise described in the chapter on intercourse (p. 255). Sometimes, for example, the woman simply requires additional foreplay or time to reach the peak of the arousal curve.

Likewise, some women require additional stimulation of the clitoris to achieve orgasm, and some sexual positions don't allow for proper clitoral stimulation. This can be easily corrected if the woman rubs her pelvis against the man during intercourse, or if either the man or the woman massages the clitoris during vaginal intercourse. If you're concerned that such manipulation of the clitoris constitutes masturbation, you need not worry. Masturbation is the stimulation of the genitals done in place of, or in opposition to, the uniting or life-giving aspects of intercourse. Manual stimulation of the clitoris during vaginal intercourse by either the husband or the wife herself is not masturbation. These simple techniques can help a woman progress more rapidly along the arousal curve and increase her likelihood of achieving climax.

Having considered a possible mechanical cause of anorgasmia, let's examine some of the psychological or relationship issues that contribute to the inhibited ability to achieve orgasm.

A Repressive Sexual Preparation

Repressive sexual preparation is the most common reason for sexual problems among those who were virgins when they got married, though this reason is a contributing factor for others as well. Many otherwise well-meaning parents make a serious mistake by either explicitly or implicitly teaching their children to be ashamed of their sexuality. Even in homes that pay lip service to the goodness of sex after marriage, many parents fail to teach their young people *why* sex after marriage is good, concentrating only (or at least much more) on why sex *before* marriage is bad. These approaches to the sexual education of minors are strongly discouraged by the Pontifical Council for the Family document *The Truth and Meaning of Human Sexuality.* (For a friendly, Catholic guide for parents on the sexual education of children, see my book *Beyond the Birds and Bees.*) Regardless, under such limited and punitive circumstances, the young person learns to control his or her sexuality by saying, "Only bad people do this and feel this way." Over the years, this belief can become so ingrained — even unconsciously — that the person struggles to understand how a mere piece of paper (i.e., a marriage license) can absolve them of the "badness," shame, and awkwardness they feel about their sexuality. In the words of one woman I counseled:

"It was like, yesterday this was a mortal sin, and today it's supposedly a wonderful thing. But I still feel the same inside. I didn't change, and I'm not sure what did. A little bit of holy water, a few prayers, and suddenly everything's okay. I believe it in my head, but I guess it just seems a little too magical for it to make sense in my heart."

If this incomplete lesson is combined with a general awkwardness on the parents' part when it comes to discussing sexual topics, the situation is made that much worse. While the young woman raised in this environment may intellectually acknowledge sex as good (and she may have even eagerly anticipated it before marriage), she will feel an irrationally negative gut reaction to actual sexual experiences, a reaction that can make it next to impossible to enjoy the freedom necessary to fully experience the marital embrace. Each sexual encounter is then experienced as "a failure," and these "failures" pile up over time, causing the woman's frustration and resentment to increase, as lovemaking becomes "that thing that was never that good anyway and causes me to feel like an idiot every time I try to do it."

Treatment of this problem usually involves some combination of fostering an emotional connection to the truth about the goodness of the client's sexuality, routing out the irrational thoughts that undermine sexual confidence and intimacy, working through the guilt and trauma of these perceived "failures," and giving the client the tools to overcome the visceral reaction that holds him or her back from the fullness of sexual intimacy.

Guilt Due to Past Promiscuity

Many people who were very sexually liberal previous to marriage are often surprised to find that in marriage they are incapable of celebrating their sexual relationship to the fullest; this can include problems with achieving climax. This is because they're suffering from what I call eroticism poisoning. While enjoyable in the beginning, eroticism (sex that is neither unitive nor procreative and has pleasure as its only goal) causes much pain and anxiety. By making you feel more and more like an object, eroticism first causes an irrational suspicion of your own sexuality; then it makes you hypersensitive to the possibility of being used by another as a sexual object even in the presence of an otherwise loving, respectful, godly spouse. If the sexually repressed virgin can't climax in marriage because "I will be bad if I enjoy this too much," the now-faithful person who had a checkered sexual past says, "I am bad because I enjoyed this too much before, so I have to make up for my sins by not enjoying it now."

In *The Magician's Nephew*, C. S. Lewis describes a wonderful scene in which Aslan has planted the apple tree that is supposed to keep Narnia safe from the White Witch. But then the Witch plucks an apple from the tree and eats it. The children ask Aslan how the tree is supposed to work since the Witch obviously had no problem picking and eating the fruit. Aslan replies, "This is how it is for those who pick and eat the fruit at the wrong time and in the wrong way. The fruit is good, but they learn to loathe it ever after."

While Lewis was not necessarily writing about sexual pleasure, his point applies here. The more we indulge in eroticism before marriage, the more difficult it is to relate to and enjoy Holy Sex.

Recovery from this problem requires working through the issues I identified in the above section, as well as overcoming the guilt and woundedness from past painful sexual memories. Most people would understandably prefer to bury the past and pretend it can't hurt them now, but our present beliefs are at least colored, if not defined, by the sum of our past experiences. Only by overcoming the fear of facing a sinful past can we open ourselves up to the grace which will allow us to emerge from our sexual tomb and celebrate the intimacy God created us for.

Undisclosed Marital Problems

Many people who call me are initially concerned about a problem in their sexual relationship but quickly discover that the root of that problem is in unresolved, or even undisclosed, *marital* conflict. As the *Journal of Sex and Marital Therapy* has shown, the body of professional research supports the idea that poor marital communication patterns are the chief culprit in Female Orgasmic Disorder.

A healthy sexual relationship cannot flourish in the presence of disrespect, cruel humor, unmet emotional needs, or unresolved conflict. Neither can it flourish if a couple isn't comfortable enough with each other to say out loud what they need from the other to be sexually satisfied. It's not true that a marriage must be perfect for a couple to be sexually happy, but a couple must at least try their hardest to be communicative, respectful, and responsive to each other at all times. If this is not happening, one or both partners will unconsciously begin withdrawing or withholding in the sexual relationship as an automatic defense against being used by an insensitive mate. If the sexual relationship is to improve, the couple will need to work through the marital issues that are choking it off.

Sexual Trauma and Psychological Disorders

A person's enjoyment of marital sexuality will be grossly diminished by having experienced rape, sexual abuse, or other sexual trauma. Likewise, other more common psychological problems like clinical depression, anxiety disorders, obsessive-compulsive disorder, and even spiritual disorders such as lust or scrupulosity will negatively affect the quality of the sexual experience. When these problems exist, often the sexual relationship will improve spontaneously as the clinical or pastoral issues are resolved. Professional help is almost always indicated in situations such as these.

SHOULD YOU LIE?

When a woman client is struggling with anorgasmia, she will often ask me if it's ever appropriate for her to fake orgasm. In a word, no. The sexual relationship is much too sacred to be desecrated with lies, even ones told for good intentions. If a woman is tempted to lie about orgasm, that can often mean that she may either have difficulty articulating her needs in the relationship overall, or that her husband has difficulty listening to her needs when she articulates them. The temptation to lie during sex may reveal the marital problem that contributes to the difficulties with achieving climax. In other words, what else do you lie about in your marriage? Seek professional marital counseling help to overcome the problems. Resist the temptation to demean yourself, your husband, and the sacredness of the marriage bed by lying.

A WORD ABOUT MARITAL AIDS

In our foreplay chapter, in the section on touch, we briefly discussed marital aids. Marital aids, such as vibrators, can be used by a couple as part of foreplay, in order to help the woman "catch up" with her husband on the arousal curve. They may also be used to help her achieve climax in instances where the man has already climaxed and he is simply unable to continue vaginal intercourse. That said, the cautions I stated earlier apply here. You may never use these devices for masturbation, which is a selfish and isolating act. Likewise, don't allow these devices to stop you from doing the work you need to do to achieve the level of intimacy and communication that would allow you to resolve the issues that stop you and your husband from harmonizing your mutual progression along the arousal curve. Intimacy, not props, must be the source of sexual pleasure. If a marital aid can enhance your ability to attend to each other or assist you in working through a sexual problem, and if it doesn't violate the One Rule or the Four Pleasure Principles, you are free to use the marital aid. But be careful never to let it become a substitute for your mate, or the intimacy and communication required for Infallible Loving and Holy Sex.

CLAIM YOUR RIGHT

The Church teaches that both husband and wife have a right to experience the fullness of their sexual relationship. Sexual problems, because they stand at the heart of the sacrament of your marriage, should be dealt with seriously and faithfully. Stay hopeful, know that there are answers, and seek the help you need to celebrate the marriage God is calling you to have.

17 COMMON SEXUAL PROBLEMS FOR MEN

I beg pardon from Brother Ass.
— St. Francis of Assisi, repenting of the anger
he felt toward his body

"It's so embarrassing," says Ray, thirty-five, married to Jean for ten years. "I've never been able to last more than a minute or two once I'm inside Jean. She tried to be understanding at first, but anymore, sex is a total drag for her. She's fed up, and I'm humiliated. I just don't know what's wrong with me."

• • •

Frank, forty-six, married to Liz for eighteen years, explained his reason for calling me. "I just can't get it up. I used to be able to go like gangbusters. But this is crazy. Now I can't even make love to Liz once. I knew getting older would affect me, but, geez, I never knew it would be like this."

Aside from low desire, premature ejaculation and erectile dysfunction are the two most common sexual complaints affecting men. This chapter will examine common causes and moral treatments for these disorders.

PREMATURE EJACULATION

Officially, this disorder is defined as "ejaculation that occurs before it is desired." Generally speaking, however, premature ejaculation (PE) usually involves climax within one to three minutes of initiating vaginal intercourse.

The primary cause of PE is poor harmonization of the sexual arousal curve. Conventional sexologists actually agree with religious nuts like myself that young men often inadvertently train themselves to climax too

291

quickly through masturbation — especially in adolescence. The fear of being caught causes teens to rush to climax as quickly as possible. This trains the body's physiological arousal curve to go from 0 to 10 in . . . well, under one to three minutes of initiating vaginal intercourse. There are no reliable medical treatments for PE. There is however a very reliable cure that works 98 percent of the time — often within two weeks of initiating treatment, according to a body of sexology research going back to the 1950s.

The cure for PE involves resetting the body's timing along the lines of what we described in the harmonization exercise in our chapter on intercourse (p. 255). In addition to the suggestions contained in that chapter, classic treatments include the *counting* technique and the *stop-and-squeeze* technique.

The counting technique involves identifying your arousal levels and associated behavioral cues at each point from 0 (no arousal) to 10 (orgasm). Secular sex therapists often encourage clients to learn this technique through masturbation, but this is wrongheaded. Aside from the moral problems, the point of overcoming PE is harmonization with your spouse, not achieving some ideal in your own head. Doing this exercise with your spouse will not only increase the duration of your arousal cycle; it will improve sexual communication between you and your wife.

To use the counting technique with your spouse, employ the following steps. During foreplay and early intercourse, don't allow yourself to go over what you consider to be a 7 or 8 (9 represents "the point of no return") until your wife gives you a clear indication that she is near climax herself — at which point you may proceed to your own orgasm. If you find you're reaching an 8 on your scale, ask your wife to stop stimulating you, or withdraw for about thirty seconds or so, while you continue to manually or orally stimulate your wife. Once you have returned to a 5 or 6, re-initiate intercourse.

The second technique, the *stop-and-squeeze* technique, involves first learning the counting technique as described above. Next, if you find that you have difficulty stopping yourself from going past a 7, you or your wife should squeeze your penis with the thumb, forefinger and middle finger either at the very base of the penis or right under the head of the penis. Squeezing either of these areas in this manner will decrease your arousal and allow you to continue lovemaking with greater control.

As I stated, by using these techniques *with your spouse,* you can resolve your PE issues within a matter of a few weeks.

Here's one other point to consider while you're learning to use these techniques well. If you do climax earlier than you desire during intercourse, a simple solution can be to *have sex again* as soon as you can achieve an erection. (You may either continue to stimulate your wife or take a break, as she prefers). Because of the differences in the arousal curve between men and women, each time a man climaxes, it takes *longer* for him to climax — and less time for her — in subsequent instances of lovemaking.

If you find you still have difficulty with PE after attempting these methods on your own, contact the Pastoral Solutions Institute for professional assistance.

ERECTILE DYSFUNCTION

It may surprise many readers to know that men and women continue to desire and have sex throughout all the stages of adulthood, well into old age. While there is a natural decrease in the hardness of a man's erections as he ages, and although erectile dysfunction (ED), traditionally known as impotence, is a common problem among men of a certain age, it is neither inevitable nor typical.

ED may be caused by medical problems such as the hardening or blockage of blood vessels in the penis. In this case, it may be a warning sign of more serious circulatory or heart problems. Always consult your doctor when dealing with ED.

ED may also be caused by psychological and relational factors. Unlike getting aroused in the first place, maintaining an erection actually requires some degree of concentration. If a man is anxious about his performance for any reason, or resentful toward his wife, these issues may affect his ability to maintain rigidity of the penis. Furthermore, a survey of the relevant professional literature shows that low self-esteem, depression, and other psychosocial problems can cause ED.

Unless you live under a rock, you've been bombarded with spam e-mails and other information about drugs to treat ED. These drugs can be helpful, but because of their side effects, they should never be the first treatment of choice. Studies have also shown that when ED is caused by relational factors, the use of medications can actually make things worse, because the increased availability of sex only draws attention to the fact that the couple can't stand each other!

Having ruled out serious medical causes, there are several things you and your wife can do to attempt to overcome ED on your own before trying medication. First, as always, make sure your emotional and spiritual intimacy is solid. Following the recommendations made in the social intercourse section of this book will help you overcome relational concerns before they become serious problems that can affect sexual performance. Second, assuming that your relationship is in good shape, increase the intensity of foreplay. Men with mild ED may still be able to achieve an erection through more intense manual or oral stimulation. Once erect, you can continue with vaginal intercourse. Additionally, don't be intimidated if your penis is only semi-erect. Sometimes the penis will "remember" what to do if you place it inside the vagina and continue to be otherwise affectionate with your wife.

If the cause of ED is not so much relational as personal or emotional, group therapy can actually be more effective than medication. Psychiatric researchers at the University of São Paulo in Brazil assigned four hundred men with ED to various treatment groups (therapy, medication, suction pump). Ninety-five percent of the men in the therapy group found relief from their ED, while there was no change in the other treatment groups over the same period of time.

Of course, if all else fails, there is always the medication option, but always consult with your doctor. Never borrow pills for ED from a friend or purchase them online. These pills can have side effects, and can exacerbate an existing medical condition or interact with other prescription or over-the-counter drugs you're taking. Never use them recreationally, and never use them without direct consultation with your physician.

As an aside, some people who are on the NACWATC mailing list wonder why, since the Church doesn't approve of contraception, Catholic teaching doesn't oppose the use of medications to treat ED. The answer really should be obvious: the Church is always in favor of medical interventions that help the body act more like God made it to act. If there were a pill that increased blood flow to the vagina and improved vaginal lubrication so women could overcome painful intercourse or anorgasmia, the Church would absolutely be in favor of it. But the Church will never favor a medical intervention that treats a healthy body and normal bodily functions as a disease. That's the difference.

19 OVERCOMING INFERTILITY

Raise a glad cry, you barren one who did not bear, break forth in jubilant song, you who were not in labor. Fear not, you shall not be put to shame; you need not blush, for you shall not be disgraced. —Isaiah 54:1a, 4

Infertility affects 17 to 26 percent of all couples. It's one of the most difficult burdens a couple could be asked to bear. The longing for a child is a laudable and noble desire, but it can sometimes bring with it great psychological and relational pain. Worse, this pain can sometimes lead couples to experience a desperation that propels them to pursue parenthood by any means necessary. In this chapter, we'll explore some of the problems with conventional infertility treatments, and we'll identify healthy, permissible options for faithful couples.

Infertility is defined as the inability to achieve a sustainable pregnancy after one full year of regular, unprotected sex during the woman's fertile phase. Infertility can be "primary" if a couple has never conceived a child, or "secondary" if they've previously had children. Because achieving pregnancy can depend upon a couple knowing how to identify the different phases of a woman's cycle, often couples will learn some form of Natural Family Planning as a first line of treatment.

One of the most difficult concepts to grasp is that while children are a great and desirable blessing, no one has the "right" to a child. This sounds cruel, but it isn't. You simply can't claim a right to another person. You can claim a right to a thing—a vote, your day in court, a raise according to the terms of your contract. But you can't claim a right to a *person*.

Return with me to high school for a moment, and recall someone who had a crush on you, whose affections you did not return. What if one day that individual came to you and said, "I long for you so deeply. I think of you all day and all night. I have decided, therefore, that I have a right to you. Come along!" Worse, what if your friends and family tried to make you commit yourself to this relationship because, after all, your admirer had a longing; therefore he or she had rights over you.

You would be mortified, and rightly so. Even if some part of you was willing to go, this behavior would still feel wrong because you're being claimed as a right, not treated as a person. People cannot claim a right to possess another person, no matter how much they may long for that person. That is not love. That is not parenthood. To claim the right to acquire or possess another person, for any reason, is slavery.

In order to have a legitimate claim over another person, that person must give himself freely to you, or *be given* by the only one who has the authority to give one person to another, namely, God.

That is one of the reasons the Church objects to treatments like artificial insemination and in vitro fertilization. They treat the baby — a person — as a thing to be acquired, and a person can never be acquired by another person for even the best reasons. One person can only be given to another. One lover can *give* himself or herself to another, and a child can *be given* to the lovers. The means by which God gives lovers to each other and the lovers a baby is Holy Sex. To remove babymaking from lovemaking is to destroy the process God created by which persons are freely given to one another. And separating babymaking from lovemaking turns pregnancy into a commercial enterprise, not an act of love.

There's an appalling trend among fertility clinics to offer "get a baby or your money back" guarantees. There is simply no way to view this industry as anything but the facilitation of the buying and selling of human persons for financial gain.

This view can be hard to accept, but refusal to accept it doesn't change the facts. And there are other objections to conventional treatments for infertility. For instance, sperm counts usually require masturbation, which is problematic for the Christian. Artificial insemination often utilizes donor sperm, which intentionally robs any resulting child from ever knowing his or her biological father. While many adults who desire a baby don't think much of such concerns, we're living at a time when the first generation of children born of donor parents are coming of age, and not a small number of the 1 million donor-conceived children in the United States are beginning to ask painful questions about their paternity. A poignant article in the *New York Times* (November 20, 2005) describes the pain of several such children searching for their roots. In the words of one young woman, "I hate when people that use [donor insemination] say that biology doesn't matter [cough, *my mom*, cough]. Because if it really didn't matter to them, then why would they use D.I. at all? They could just adopt or something and help out kids in need."

The bottom line is that Christians may never do a wrong thing to achieve a good end. Never, and regardless of how they feel. Everyone who plans to do something that is wrong thinks their situation is the exception. Everyone who plans to do something wrong thinks their reasons are justifiable. It is up to the person of integrity to be willing to make the sacrifices that stand up to the face of relativism and say, "No. I want to choose options that are safe, respectful of my body, and respectful of the dignity of any child I would bring into the world."

Returning to the issue of in vitro, another problem (beyond the way it renders sex and the body as obsolete) is the issue of multiple fertilization. Couples often are encouraged to selectively murder all but one of the children conceived through artificial reproductive technologies so that the one child has a greater likelihood of being brought to term (and so that the parents won't be stressed by all the unwanted bonus babies). Couples who have been desperate to achieve pregnancy can become even more desperate to sustain a pregnancy once it's been achieved and may find themselves seriously considering things — like murder for the "greater good" of a child — they would never have believed themselves capable of.

Even if a couple would not personally engage in selective reduction, they are participating in and actively supporting an industry that sees selective abortion as the standard of care. This is a bit like saying, "I would never hire a hit man. I just use my local mafia contacts so I can play the ponies." There is never a good reason to line the pockets of those who make a living by manufacturing life in the lab and then selling it as a commodity to desperate couples.

FALSE INFORMATION ABOUT IVF SUCCESS RATES

According to the journal *Human Reproduction*, IVF (in vitro fertilization) clinics regularly manipulate their statistics to make their success rates look better than they actually are. The actual rates of success for IVF treatment are between 1 percent and 50 percent, depending upon the specific cause of the infertility. Many clinics report much higher success rates because they simply weed out, discourage, or waitlist the patients with more complex problems, and move the simplest cases to the front of the line. This allows IVF clinics to report stunning success rates while really not helping anyone but the people who need the least help — but these folks may still end up paying as much as they would if they were a more complex case. According to *Human Reproduction*, this crass behavior is standard operating procedure in infertility treatment, not just in the United States but around the world. As for those money-back guarantees I mentioned above, when you consider that many clinics will take only the people who have the easiest cases — charging them the full rate while stringing along couples with more complex cases "until there's room for them on the doctor's schedule" — this financial incentive starts looking less like a humanitarian concern for financially strapped parents and more like the mercenary marketing gimmick it is.

BUT IT'S A DISEASE!

In our discussion of erectile dysfunction, I noted that the Church approves of any medical intervention that helps the body do what it was created to do. The argument does not apply to IVF and many other artificial reproductive technologies (ART) because they do not help the body do what God made it to do. Instead, most ARTs allow doctors to do themselves what the body *ought* to do. They substitute mechanical manipulation for natural bodily processes. They take the egg out of the body, harvest sperm outside of the body, fertilize the egg in a lab outside the body, and then, once the whole process is complete, implant it in the body. This is not "helping the body do what God designed it to do by medical intervention." Rather, this is "making the body itself irrelevant in favor of artificially combining various pieces of the body so that I can create what I want to make." This is why the "curing disease" argument doesn't wash for IVF. For Christians, whose spirituality is intimately incarnational and tied up in bodiliness, rendering the body irrelevant and reducing and manipulating its component parts is hugely problematic. IVF is simply low-Church gnosticism with all its "the body doesn't matter" doctrine applied to medical ethics. Brave new world, indeed.

GOOD NEWS! THERE ARE HEALTHY OPTIONS

Fortunately, there is hope for Christians who value the incarnational reality of their faith and wish to pursue healthy, viable, morally sound options for treatment of infertility.

First of all, fertility drugs are the primary treatment for problems with ovulation, and they're an absolutely permissible means of treating this type of infertility problem, because they work with the body to enable it to do what God created it to do.

Additionally, Catholic hospitals often offer procedures that are more humane and respectful of the rights of the potential child. When evaluating problems with male fertility, moral sperm collection can be achieved by using a perforated condom during normal intercourse. This allows the act to be potentially, naturally life-giving and unitive while retaining enough of a sperm sample to be analyzed. Catholic hospitals also tend to focus on procedures that treat the root problems of infertility, such as treating ovulatory dysfunction or blockages in the fallopian tubes, or the surgical transfer of an egg, fertilized through natural intercourse, to a position below a tubal blockage. These procedures are appropriate because they do not add a third party (either doctor or donor) whose job it is to render either sex or the body afterthoughts to natural procreation. Some procedures offered at some Catholic hospitals may be questionably moral because of their superficial similarity to IVF or artificial insemination. They are offered, in some cases, because competent Church authorities have not yet determined officially whether they are permissible. Two prominent examples of these procedures are GIFT (gamete intra-fallopian transfer) and intrauterine insemination. Because couples are often presented with a dizzying array of medical and moral factors when contemplating infertility treatments, I strongly recommend that, prior to seeking treatment, you consult with the National Catholic Bioethics Center (*NcbCenter.org*), which offers telephone consultations with experts in bioethics. These competent, sensitive professionals can help couples plan effective, moral courses of action for addressing fertility issues.

THE POPE PAUL VI CENTER

An additional option for you is the Pope Paul VI Institute at Creighton University in Omaha (*PopePaulVI.com*), which offers medical and surgical options (and a national physician referral network) for couples who are struggling with infertility. Unlike conventional assisted reproductive technologies, their methods do not treat the body as an irrelevant afterthought. The Institute seeks to diagnose and cure the problems that were preventing the body from doing what God created it to do. In some cases, this can help couples achieve subsequent pregnancies naturally without further intervention (unlike IVF).

The Institute and its national network of physicians and surgeons trained in Natural Procreative Technology offer excellent success rates at a fraction of the cost of conventional ART treatment. They address infertility, repeated miscarriage, hormonal imbalances, ovulatory defects, cervical disorders, and other reproductive problems with medications, medical interventions, and surgical procedures that seek to cure the underlying causes of the problem. Couples who are seeking medically and morally sound options for the treatment of infertility and reproductive disorders should contact the Institute at *www.PopePaulVI.com* or by calling (402) 390-6600 for information, referrals, or appointments.

THE WAITING CHILD — AN ADOPTION OPTION

I would be remiss if I didn't ask infertile couples — indeed, all couples — to seriously and prayerfully consider adoption. You may not be in a place where you want to consider this option at this time, but I'm writing as an adoptive father and as someone who has been involved with foster care and adoption in one capacity or another for almost thirty years. There are many beautiful children who need your love. If you want a child, there are children waiting — for you. If you find yourself going down the path of "I must conceive a child by any means necessary," I would gently encourage you to ask yourself whether you want a child, or you just want your way. That's as hard a question to ask as it is to answer. I don't blame you for wanting what you want the way you want it. It's only human. But don't close off your options. The child God may have in mind for you may already be waiting next door, or even around the world. Give God the freedom to build the family the way that he knows is best for your family. Don't rule out adoption as a realistic and beautiful option.

TAKING CARE OF EACH OTHER

Regardless of the treatment options you pursue, infertility can be very hard on marriages. According to an article in the *Lancet,* infertile couples struggle with high rates of anxiety, depression, and impaired marital functioning. Couples have to work hard to maintain their levels of social intercourse in order to prevent their lovemaking — or for that matter, their entire marriage — from deteriorating into a perceived series of successive failures to produce a baby. Couples struggling with infertility must remember that love is the point of lovemaking, and the absence of a baby does not lessen their love or the legitimacy of the couples' sexual union.

According to research in *Family Process*, one of the factors that makes all the difference for couples struggling with infertility is cohesion; that is, the couple needs to be on the same page — emotionally speaking — regarding their desire for a child and their struggle with achieving pregnancy. Dealing with infertility is hard enough. A spouse who also feels that he or she cares about their struggle more than the other partner has an especially painful burden to bear. This is another instance where the husband and wife must love each other even better. Remember the words of St. Josemaría Escrivá, which we cited earlier:

> *God in His providence has two ways of blessing marriages: one by giving them children; and the other, sometimes, because he loves them so much, by not giving them children. I don't know which is the better blessing. In any event, let one accept his own.*

By rising to the challenges that infertility presents to you both, even as you strive to resolve your difficulties with achieving pregnancy, you can help each other become saints by perfecting each other in love. What does it profit you to gain a baby if you lose your love and your soul? Reach out to each other in genuine love and trust that the Lord has answers. Seek appropriate medical care. Take care of each other by attending to the techniques I recommend in this book and in *For Better . . . FOREVER!* for strengthening your marriage in good times and in bad. For those struggling to discern God's will in the midst of their suffering, I also encourage you to read my book *Life Shouldn't Look Like This: Dealing with Disappointment in the Light of Faith.*

20 INFIDELITY

Christ condemns even adultery of mere desire (see Matt. 5:27–28). The sixth commandment and the New Testament forbid adultery absolutely. The prophets . . . see it as an image of the sin of idolatry (see Hos. 2:7; Jer. 5:7, 13:27). Adultery is an injustice. He who commits adultery fails in his commitment. He does injury to the sign of the covenant which the marriage bond is, transgresses the rights of the other spouse, and undermines the institution of marriage. . . . He compromises the good of human generation and the welfare of children who need their parents' stable union.
  — Catechism of the Catholic Church nos. 2380–81

Adultery is a serious problem, not just from a moral perspective but from a psychological and relational perspective as well. Adultery causes incredible pain and takes a great deal of work to recover from. According to research published in the *Journal of Family Psychology*, infidelity is rated by marital therapists as the third most difficult marital problem to treat, after the complete loss of loving feelings (#1) and alcoholism (#2). It is, unfortunately, a fairly common problem. A study conducted by Catholic sociologist Rev. Andrew Greeley found that infidelity affects between 20 percent and 25 percent of all marriages.

WHAT CAUSES IT?

In very broad terms, there are two different types of infidelity — one-night stands, and affairs. One-night stands are usually caused by a trifecta of alcohol, distance, and opportunity. This is why it's so important to avoid not only romantic settings with the opposite sex while alone and away from home, but also to avoid spending too much of any kind of time alone with a member of the opposite sex, especially if alcohol is involved.

When possible, inviting a third party along to meetings with a member of the opposite sex is prudent and may save you from a world of grief.

One-night stands are difficult to recover from, but they tend to be somewhat easier to deal with than affairs because of their episodic nature and the lack of an emotional commitment. While recovery from one-night stands and affairs tends to follow the same course, affairs are much more difficult to handle.

Most people think that marital dissatisfaction causes affairs, but this is a myth. Many people have marital problems, but not all people who have marital problems go on to have affairs. That means there has to be something else causing infidelity besides unhappiness in the relationship. A 2007 study conducted by University of Colorado psychologist Dr. Mark Whisman found that when a spouse is both unhappy in a marriage and exhibits either low self-esteem or a tendency to be easily given to feelings of anger, anxiety, depression, or despair, that spouse is at significantly higher risk for having an affair. And if you add pregnancy to the mix in this dynamic, the risk of the man having an affair goes through the roof.

RELATIONSHIP AS SELF-MEDICATION

Generally speaking, the person who commits adultery (I'm referring now to affairs, not so much one-night stands, except in the case of serial offenders) is someone who's not very good at three things: (1) making their needs know in relationship; (2) following through on advocating for those needs, even if they do manage to articulate them; and (3) dealing with interpersonal conflict (curiously, this person may not have a problem with work conflict, where there is less of one's heart on the line).

Such a spouse may say to his (or her) mate, "I would really like X." But if the mate doesn't immediately jump up and down and say, "Oh, yes! That sounds like a wonderful idea!" the spouse who made the request — because he tends toward easy despair and hates conflict — will simply give up and assume that the mate doesn't care to meet his needs. The disappointed spouse usually tries to adjust by withdrawing from the relationship and trying to seek happiness at work, in hobbies, or in other social outlets. The disappointed spouse's partner may feel a little neglected, but otherwise is usually clueless to the fact that the partner is cooking up a slow-burn of hate and resentment that is poisoning the marriage.

Multiply this interaction by thousands of times over the course of several years, and the spouse who consistently gives up much and too easily begins getting depressed; he feels powerless to get any of his needs met in the marital relationship. Over time, the depression and frustration build and the spouse, who believes that the depression is his mate's fault for being so insensitive (as opposed to blaming himself for having no backbone) passive-aggressively lashes out by seeking someone else who can make him feel better. The affair is not primarily an attempt to fix or even respond to a marital problem. It's an attempt to self-medicate for the depression.

RECOVERY

When an affair is discovered, the couple often initially tries to solve the problem just by calling off the extramarital relationship, being generally nicer to each other, and going out on more regular dates. This is especially true of the offending spouse, who hates conflict anyway and certainly doesn't want to deal with it now. If the wounded spouse wishes to do other things to address the problem (counseling, marriage retreats, talking with a pastor), the offending, conflict — and vulnerability — averse spouse may raise all kinds of objections, insisting that "we just have to let it go and leave it in the past."

Here's the bad news. If this is all the couple does to address their issues, the couple runs an extraordinarily high risk of dooming the marriage either to another affair down the line, or divorce, as the wounded mate's unresolved and squelched pain festers.

Here's the good news: you can resolve the problems related to infidelity and go on to have an outstanding relationship. According to research in *The Good Marriage*, upward of 20 percent of couples who presently

306

report high levels of marital happiness have at one time in their past weathered infidelity, but it takes real work. Successfully recovering from an affair involves the following steps. (These usually require the support of a competent therapist to negotiate effectively.)

1. Ending the Affair

This is a no-brainer. All contact with the paramour has to end. The offending spouse must demonstrate a willingness to do everything possible (as determined by the wounded spouse) to put distance between himself (or herself) and the paramour.

2. Confession

I do, of course, mean sacramental Confession, but I also mean confession to the wounded spouse. The wounded spouse has a right to all the information about the affair that she (or he) wishes to have. The wounded spouse should never be put in the position of pulling information out of the cheater. The offending spouse must willingly offer all the details and information the other wishes to hear. This is because, according to a study in the *Journal in Social and Clinical Psychology*, forgiveness is absolutely essential to recovery, but the wounded spouse can't forgive what she doesn't know. Full confession is not only good for the soul; it is essential for the reconciliation of the marriage.

3. Establishment of Basic Rapport

In this step, the couple works hard on their marriage. They must work to create a marriage that is far better than they have ever experienced before. They must completely overhaul their social intercourse and commit to the kind of intimacy, communication, and attentiveness facilitated by such activities as the Daily Marital Checkup Exercise (p. 213), the establishment of a greater number and frequency of bonding rituals and routines (p. 210), the social intercourse variation of the Lovelist Exercise (p. 214; not the Sexual Lovelist Exercise, since the couple may not be ready to resume a sexual relationship for a while), and other activities like those described in *For Better...FOREVER!* or prescribed by the couple's counselor.

This work is essential because the couple — especially the wounded spouse — must be able to see a real, sustained, and substantively different amount of effort being applied to the relationship if they are ever to be able to move on. Returning to the way things were before is not an option because the wounded spouse believed everything was fine then. If things just go back to the way they were, the wounded spouse will always feel an unconscious suspicion that won't go away. In order to overcome the suspicion, the marriage can't be just like it was. It must become better than it has ever been.

4. The Offending Spouse Must Address Personal Problems

This is the hardest step. The offending spouse, being conflict-avoidant and fearing vulnerability, just wants to have a superficially happy relationship and ignore his or her hatred of conflict and tendencies toward neuroticism (this is the technical term for the tendency of the offending spouse to become easily offended and bury the emotional pain). This approach is doomed. Remember, it was these personality problems and not the couple's marital problems that caused the affair in the first place. If the couple had only marital problems, they would simply have worked out their problems directly. But because the offending spouse didn't know — and still doesn't know — how to address disappointment and frustrations directly, the couple remains at high risk for repeating the cycle in the future, regardless of what the offending spouse might say today.

The offending spouse will need to learn to open up, communicate and problem-solve more effectively, and overcome his or her fears of emotional vulnerability if the couple hopes to do more than just get by. Additionally, as the Whisman study found, sincere religious involvement tends to make marriages affair-resistant. This is for two reasons. First, the sincerely religious person takes moral prohibitions against infidelity much more seriously than others do. Second, sincere religious faith requires *vulnerability*.

Getting the offending spouse to become active in his or her faith is an excellent way to support the other therapeutic work that must be done.

5. Overcoming Irrational Fears, Doubts, and Guilt That Remain

Even after the marriage is better than ever, and the offending spouse is more open and competent at conflict management and more vulnerable than ever, lingering doubts may still remain in the wounded spouse, and persistent feelings of unworthiness and guilt may afflict the offending spouse. The couple may need the benefit of cognitive therapy strategies to help them learn how to evaluate and resolve these irrational and undesirable emotional roadblocks to full recovery.

HEALING IS POSSIBLE

As I mentioned at the outset, making a full recovery from infidelity is certainly possible, but it is never a do-it-yourself project. Infidelity is marital cancer that requires competent, multi-stage, multi-modal treatment by a marriage-friendly therapist. To learn what to seek in a therapist, review chapter 22 in this book titled "When to Seek Help," or contact the Pastoral Solutions Institute (*www.exceptionalmarriages.com*) to arrange for marital telecounseling with pastoral counselors who have been trained in the methods outlined in this chapter. Additionally, organizations such as Retrouvaille can offer peer support as an adjunct (though never a replacement) to competent marital counseling.

Regardless of where you turn for help, know that there is healing for your injured heart and troubled marriage. Faithfully work at the recovery tasks in front of you, and trust that the Lord will guide you to the peace and wholeness that is your right to expect from your marriage.

21 MASTURBATION AND PORNOGRAPHY

A man who governs his passions is master of the world. We must either command them or be enslaved by them. It is better to be a hammer than an anvil. — St. Dominic

Imagine that you inherit a great treasure. The treasure is so wonderful that you become fascinated with it. In fact, you become so fascinated with it that you decide to keep it all to yourself.

If you persist in this relationship with your treasure, what will you become?

My Precious . . .

Some readers will catch the Tolkien allusion above. Golem, the hobbit who became fascinated with his "precious" (the One Ring), loved it more than anything and anyone and let his disordered love turn him into a monster incapable of loving anything but the thing that could never give him any real satisfaction.

The crew from NACWATC would have you believe that Catholics think of masturbation as a sin because, again, the silly men in pointy hats hate pleasure. By now, you know this is a myth. Catholics assert that masturbation is a sin because it makes a person take the incredible treasure that is sexual intimacy and horde it for themselves. Masturbation is not a sin because it is pleasurable. It is a sin because it is not pleasurable enough. Creating good feelings is great, but it is much, much greater to create good feelings with a person who loves you in the context of a relationship that is so awesome it has the power to bring new life into the world. God wants to give us the banquet at the Ritz-Carlton, and the masturbator wants to say, "No thanks. I'll just go visit the dumpster around back."

The *Catechism of the Catholic Church* (no. 2352) puts it this way: "[With masturbation] pleasure is sought outside of the sexual relationship . . . in which the total meaning of mutual self-giving and human procreation in the context of true love is achieved."

In the original 2002 *Spider-Man* film, we are told (over and over and over) that "with great power comes great responsibility." The maxim, clichéd though it may be, resonates because *it happens to be true*. Infallible Lovers know that masturbation is an irresponsible use of the power of the gift that could otherwise be Holy Sex. It takes the impulse that should be allowed to grow into Holy Sex, strips it bare, and hordes it all for oneself until Golem ends up sleeping in your bed (*eeew!*).

There is a notion that masturbation is fine because it's done in private and for one's own pleasure. This statement always struck me as a little absurd. Suppose someone said to you, "Having a few drinks at a party can be fun, but getting sloshed alone is even better. After all, so long as it's done in private and for my own pleasure, what's the harm?" Most people would think the person who made such a claim was odd at best, and more than a little sad. Now, imagine that same person writing a book called *The Joys of Drinking Alone*, and moreover, imagine that book being reviewed in the *New York Times Review of Books* as "a taboo-breaking homage to one man's brave love for solitary boozing." Crazy, huh? Except that's exactly what has happened to masturbation. It has gone from being viewed with suspicion by religious and secular people alike (Freud had especially harsh things to say about it at one point) to being something that people are applauded for admitting they are addicted to, as they publish how-to manuals to convert other potential addicts.

FIVE ARGUMENTS FROM PSYCHOLOGY

No doubt, there are those who remain unconvinced, so allow me to examine the psychology of masturbation. At a conference on psychology and religion, New York University professor emeritus and author Paul Vitz articulated five secular arguments against masturbation. I build on those arguments and offer them for your consideration here.

1. Masturbation Is Narcissistic

In his book *Authentic Happiness,* University of Pennsylvania psychologist and happiness researcher Martin Seligman argues that authentic happiness is rooted in becoming more intimate and engaged with others. By contrast, the more self-involved you are, the shallower, and ultimately the less happy, you become. Masturbation takes something that should be a path to sanctification and communion with others and turns it into a miserly act that is all about keeping the gift to oneself. In this sense, masturbation is contrary not just to healthy morality, but to the pursuit of authentic happiness itself.

2. Masturbation Is Regressive

As Dr. Vitz puts it, as far as a self-comforting strategy, masturbation is "one step above thumb sucking." People who masturbate habitually often do it as a way of dealing with the stress that comes from problems in life. But grown-ups deal with the problems of life by facing them and solving them, not by retreating to a dark room with a glowing screen and a box of tissues.

3. Masturbation Is Addictive

Masturbation artificially stimulates the pleasure centers of the brain and releases the bonding chemicals that accompany sexual release. Although the biochemical bonding impulse is engaged, there is, however, nothing to bond to — except the act itself. This is why the more a person masturbates, the more they want to masturbate, until they feel that they have a need to masturbate or they begin to get irritable. This is not unlike what happens when a person withdraws from any other addictive substance.

4. Masturbation Is Objectifying

Masturbation turns people into objects in two ways. First, masturbation is usually accompanied by the use of pornography (discussed below). Masturbation is the sole reason pornography exists. It's the sole reason millions of women are treated like things that can be posed and thrown away instead of people who have a right to be loved. There are those who say that pornography is acceptable because the "models" seem to be enjoying themselves or, in some cases, publicly claim to enjoy themselves. This argument tends to assume that the women who pose for pornography belong to "that group of people over there who like that sort of thing." But they are just people like you and me. Sit with that a moment and then ask yourself what it would take — what you would have to go through — before you would be willing to allow yourself to be photographed in that manner. Would you have to have been told that all you had to offer the world was your looks and your sex? Would you have to have had your sexual boundaries violated sufficiently that you lost all sense of modesty and the desire not to be used by others? What would it take? That's what it took for those women there too — and worse. If you don't believe me, all you have to do is look at the rates of drug and alcohol abuse, eating disorders, plastic surgery addictions, "cutting," and other self-destructive behaviors engaged in by pornography "stars," and you'll see the glamour of evil for what it truly is.

The second sense in which masturbation is objectifying is that it teaches the person who masturbates to think that real people should act just like the models in the images, or (when pornography is not used) that real people exist to simply scratch the individual's sexual itch. A personal side effect of objectifying others is that masturbation can damage the person's ability to harmonize their arousal curve with that of their spouse (see the section on premature ejaculation, p. 291 above).

5. Masturbation Is Progressive

Like any addiction, eventually you need more of it, and more extreme forms of it, to maintain the chemical high achieved by the behavior. People who habitually masturbate need more intense stimuli (new forms of pornography, toys, etc.) to keep up the same level of chemical well-being artificially created by the masturbatory act. As will become clear in our discussion of online pornography and sexual addiction, under the right circumstances, a person can come to prefer masturbation to almost any other activity. This sounds ridiculous, but addictions are ridiculous. That's what makes them addictions!

CUT THAT OUT!

I have purposefully avoided much discussion of the moral claims against masturbation because I wanted to demonstrate that a case can be made, mainly from psychology and neuroendocrinology, that masturbation is what the Catholic Church says it is, a distortion of the sexual act that can destroy the person — that is what is meant by the phrase "mortal sin." Even so, I would be remiss in failing to mention the scriptural data opposing the practice. As you know from our discussion of the contraception question, masturbation is condemned in the Old Testament in the story of Onan (Gen. 38:4). Jewish and Christian scholars from antiquity until the most recent times have all but universally interpreted this passage as a twin condemnation of both contraception and masturbation. What you may not know is that tradition holds that Jesus also condemned lust and masturbation in his famous speech in Matthew 18:8–9.

> *If your hand or foot causes you to sin, cut it off and throw it away. It is better for you to enter into life maimed or crippled than to be thrown into eternal fire. And if your eye causes you to sin, tear it out and throw it away. It is better for you to enter into life with one eye than with two eyes to be thrown into fiery Gehenna.*

How is this a condemnation of masturbation? In Aramaic, the language Jesus spoke, the word "foot" was used as a euphemism/pun for the penis. Puts that passage in a rather different light, doesn't it?

Now, before any of you latter-day Origens are tempted to reenact his famous episode of self-castration, just step away from the knife and let's talk. Pleasure isn't bad. But pleasure is only good when it is sought in the right way at the right time in the right context. To do less is to allow yourself to settle for less than you deserve and risk your ability to receive all

God wishes to give you: truly healthy, whole, and holy sexual intimacy with a person who loves you freely, fruitfully, faithfully, and forever. Despite what the shills at NACWATC tell you, victory over lust is possible. You can, in the words of that great philosopher-king Jerry Seinfeld, learn to "master your domain," and the great news is that you don't even have to cut anything off to do it. Because masturbation is so often tied to the use of pornography, however, I will present some of those strategies in the following sections.

PORNOGRAPHY AND SEXUAL ADDICTION

It used to be that only we religious nuts (as well as the odd secular feminist) would shriek about the dangers of pornography, while the rest of popular culture would pat us on the head and smile, the way you do with the crazy uncle who visits once a year so you just have to put up with him.

Then along came the Internet. And the secular world has had to wake up to the massive numbers of collapsed marriages and lost hours of employee productivity caused by easy access to porn. Even secular counselors, long the High Priests of Prurient Interests, have had to realize that the overturning of too many cultural taboos might not be such a good thing after all. According to the *Psychotherapy Networker*, secular treatment programs for online sexual addiction are now a multimillion-dollar business.

Better late than never, I suppose.

How Big Is the Problem?

Studies show that about 10 percent of all computer users admit to engaging in compulsive online behavior that seriously jeopardizes work or important social relationships.

According to research published in the journal *Sexual Addiction and Compulsivity*, 56 billion dollars a year is spent on masturbatory media. This is a shocking amount of money. How shocking? According to figures produced by the World Bank, the amount of money spent on masturbatory media worldwide is greater than the Gross Domestic Product of all but 55 of the 183 nation-states belonging to the International Monetary Fund. Think of the healthcare, famine relief, schools, and other social services that could be provided for the same amount of money people spend on the porn industry, and then ask again why the Church considers masturbation a mortal sin.

Cybersex addicts spend an estimated fifteen to twenty-five hours a week online viewing sexual material. That's the equivalent of a part-time job. When you consider that some studies demonstrate that parents, on average, spend no more than fifteen minutes a day in direct, face-to-face interactions with their children (and often complain they simply don't have time to do more), you get a sense of the massive amount of time and energy directed at cybersex.

What Is Addiction?

Addiction may be understood as the uncontrolled and compulsive use of a substance or indulgence in an activity. Addiction is uncontrolled in the sense that persons suffering from an addiction can't stop themselves from using the addictive substance or participating in the destructive activity even when they sincerely promise they will. Sometimes, a person suffering from addiction is unable to stop even after suffering serious personal consequences.

Likewise, addiction is compulsive in the sense that while addicts feel the irresistible need to engage in the addictive behavior, they get less and less pleasure from the addiction as time passes. People with an addiction problem eventually derive little pleasure from it, may experience negative consequences for it, and usually hate themselves for being unable to stop it.

Characteristics of the Addict

The frightening truth is that anyone, young or old, well-educated or not, rich or poor, even male or female, can become addicted to pornography. There are certain factors that increase a person's likelihood of such addiction. Earlier — in our review of the Fourth Power of Holy Sex — we observed the basic human need to feel connected. Attachment scientists tell us there are many ways a person can experience this sense of connectedness to others: spiritual, emotional, social (e.g., a sense of belonging), psychological (through identification with a person), and through the senses. Of these, the last type of connection, sensory connectedness, is the weakest, because it is chemically based. When the chemistry washes out of the system, the sense of connection evaporates. If a person's capacity for spiritual, emotional, social, or psychological connection is impaired or absent, the person is forced to lean more and more heavily on sensory connection to make up the difference. In intimate relationships, this means a greater and greater reliance on sex. But no one — not even the couple with the healthiest libido — can have sex all the time, so what happens to the person who, because of an impaired ability to connect on some or all of the other levels, must rely more heavily on a sensory connection? He (or she) has to find some other way to simulate the sense of chemical connectedness to bridge the gap.

The more people struggle to make connections with others on the spiritual, emotional, social, or psychological level, the more they will lean on their senses to feel connected, and the more they may ultimately feel they need pornography and masturbation to bridge the gap between the times when a flesh-and-blood person is there. In fact, it's well known that pornography is a "gateway drug" to more risky sexual behavior with other people. As time goes by, the images just don't cut it any more. The addict needs more three-dimensional stimuli (dolls, people) to trick the body into feeling the same level of sensory connection that images once delivered.

Exercise

SEXUAL ADDICTION:
DO YOU HAVE A PROBLEM?

The website *UnityRestored.com* is an excellent resource for men and women who would like to learn more about the effect of pornography on their lives and relationships. Here are some questions UnityRestored asks to help visitors determine whether they need help overcoming a budding (or full-blown) addiction to pornography. Answer "Yes" or "No" to each of the following questions:.

_____ Are you using the Internet more frequently or for a longer time for sex-related activities?

_____ Are you spending less time with your spouse and kids or other people?

_____ Are you becoming less productive in your work (because of time spent surfing for porn)?

_____ Do you feel that you need to view more (or more intense) pornography? (This could be a symptom of tolerance.)

_____ When you don't use porn, do you experience anxiety, difficulty concentrating, or restlessness and unease? (These could be symptoms of withdrawal.)

_____ Are you growing increasingly more obsessed with viewing pornographic images?

_____ Have you failed to stop viewing (or you stop for a while, only to start up again) — despite adverse consequences to personal health, career, significant relationships, or spiritual life?

If you answered "Yes" to any one of these questions, you may be experiencing an addiction to pornography. The more affirmative answers you give, the stronger the hold pornography has on you.

Getting Help

Overcoming an addiction — even an addiction to masturbation or pornography — always involves more than simply stopping your association with the addictive substance or activity. Perhaps you've heard the phrase "dry drunk"? A dry drunk is someone who doesn't drink anymore but still maintains the irresponsible, narcissistic, isolating, and unreliable ways of life that accompany alcoholism. The sexually compulsive "dry drunk" will continue to struggle with an inability to make spiritual, emotional, social, and psychological connection with others even if the masturbatory materials are eliminated. Chances are that they are also not very good at making their needs known to others and swallow a lot of frustration and resentment rather than working it out. Pornography addiction may also cause changes to the actual structure and chemistry of the brain. Until the pornography addict addresses these issues, he or she can't be free of the addiction. The following are some types of therapy that, depending upon the severity and nature of the problem, may help.

Self-Help for Masturbation and Pornography Addiction

There are good self-help strategies for you if you struggle with masturbation and pornography addiction.

First, the more you struggle with the impulse to masturbate or use pornography, the more you must pour yourself into seeking greater spiritual, emotional, social, and psychological connections with the actual people with whom you share your life. When the temptation to masturbate or use pornography strikes, understand that this is your body's way of telling you it's craving *connection,* but you have taught it to rely too heavily on sensory connection to the exclusion of stronger forms of attachment. Focus on the suggestions made earlier in this book for improving your capacity for social intercourse. It doesn't matter whether or not you think you are doing enough in these areas. You will know you are doing "enough" when the desire to masturbate or use porn decreases to resistible levels.

Second, you must reconnect your sexual impulse with its godly purpose. As we discussed earlier in this book, God's intention for creating sexual attraction was to remind us that it is not good for us to be alone and to draw us closer to others so that we can identify ways we can be a gift to them. If you struggle with masturbation or pornography, you have turned an impulse that is supposed to make us *more* generous and turned it into a miserly, selfish, objectifying impulse. Self-help strategies involve identifying the earliest moment of the addictive impulse (about a 3 or 4 on the 10 point arousal curve we discussed earlier), remembering that the point of the impulse is not to use others or indulge yourself but rather to serve others. Then throw yourself totally into a specific action that demonstrates love, caring, service, and support for a real person in your life. This method uses simple behavioral conditioning strategies (classical conditioning) to pair the sexual impulse with intentional, loving service. For individuals whose addiction has not progressed to a significant degree, this can be an important way to retrain the sexual impulse to do what God made it to do — make you a more generous, loving, and connected person. If self-help strategies aren't sufficient, the following resources may be helpful.

Individual Therapy

Individual therapy for the person who struggles with chronic masturbation or pornography addiction may consist of three components:

1. Helping the person overcome compulsive tendencies caused by changes to the structure and chemistry of the brain.

The pornography addict or sexual compulsive may experience similar feelings as persons with obsessive-compulsive disorder, such as compulsive hand-washing and "checking" behaviors. They experience a repetitive, irresistible urge to indulge in a behavior that gives them momentary relief but no long-term pleasure (and in many cases, increased stress). In our tele-counseling work with sexually addicted clients through the Pastoral Solutions Institute, we have successfully used OCD treatment protocols such as Jeffrey Schwartz's Four Steps method (see his *Brain Lock: Free Yourself from Obsessive-Compulsive Behavior*) for helping clients break the addictive cycle that can become hardwired into the brain. These methods can be helpful for clients who have become dependent upon pornography in their lives.

2. Helping the client explore and overcome traumatic experiences that create barriers to authentic intimacy.

People do not deny themselves spiritual, emotional, social, or psychological connectedness with others unless they feel they have good cause. The reason clients often give for not connecting is that they are wounded on these levels. In some cases, the wounding might be that they were never taught to relate to others on these levels. Individual therapy can address these dimensions of interpersonal attachment.

3. Helping the client explore and overcome irrational thoughts related to spiritual, emotional, social, and psychological connectedness.

Many clients have convinced themselves that connecting to others on anything other than a sensual level is dangerous, undesirable, or impossible for them. Individual therapy can help clients overcome these self-limiting irrational beliefs about attachment to others.

Group Therapy

No one can challenge the addict to face the responsibilities of recovery like fellow addicts can. That's why groups like Sexaholics Anonymous (*www.sa.org*) or Sex Addicts Anonymous (*www.saa-recovery.org*) and private therapy groups focusing on overcoming sexual addiction can be a helpful, even necessary, component for recovery.

Marital Counseling

Spouses often feel they are to blame for their partners' addiction to pornography or struggle with masturbation. "This wouldn't happen if I were more attractive/more sexually adventurous/more sexually available." This is not true. The person addicted to porn becomes addicted because of *his or her own limitations* regarding conflict resolution and spiritual, emotional, social, and psychological connection. Recovery can't occur until the addicted spouse accepts primary responsibility for overcoming these problems.

Even so, marital counseling can be very useful for providing additional accountability for the addicted person, providing greater opportunities to learn authentic intimacy, overcoming unhealthy communication patterns that make intimacy seem unsafe in the marriage, offering the offended spouse support, and giving the offended spouse ways to support the addict.

Spiritual Direction

Addicts tend to struggle with seeing deeper meanings in life and relationships. Competent spiritual direction can help clients identify and connect with that deeper meaning through instruction in prayer and discernment, encouraging greater participation in the sacramental life, spiritual reading, coaching, and support.

Recovery Is Possible

There are those who would tell you that being a sexual miser and hoarding the gift of your sexuality is the most natural and wonderful thing in the world. There are those who would tell you that sexual miserliness is actually a virtue and that "denying yourself" is simply wrong. Don't believe the myths. When you masturbate, when you use pornography — that is when you are truly denying yourself the opportunity to experience true love.

It can take work, but it is absolutely worth doing the work necessary for reclaiming the godly intention of sexual desire: the intention to propel you toward greater generosity and commitment to working for the good of the people who share your life — the commitment to experience and inspire authentic love.

22 WHEN TO SEEK HELP (AND FROM WHOM)

We must endure and persevere if we are to attain the truth and freedom we have been allowed to hope for. Faith and hope are the very meaning of our being Christians, but if faith and hope are to bear fruit, patience is necessary. — St. Cyprian

There may come a time in your sexual relationship, or relationship as a whole, when you and your spouse are experiencing conflicts that you simply don't know how to resolve. These problems may be simpler issues related to disagreements about frequency, the appropriateness of certain sexual positions or practices, or discernment of whether it's time to add another child to the family. Or these issues could be more complex, for example, when your spouse is openly hostile to the importance of integrating your faith life with your sexual relationship or suggests sexual practices that you believe are degrading or objectively immoral, or if disagreements about a sexual issue are spilling over into your daily life and causing strain on your marriage.

Counseling is probably indicated if you agree with any of the following statements.

_____ Our sexual problems persist despite my spouse's and my efforts to resolve them.

_____ My spouse is hostile to integrating my (our) faith with our sexual relationship.

_____ My spouse persists in his (her) desire to engage in sexual acts that I find offensive or morally objectionable.

_____ My spouse (or I) experiences persistent sexual fantasies that are degrading or immoral.

323

_____ Despite our best efforts to resolve sexual disputes charitably, our discussions always end in arguments or resentment.

_____ Although it has caused problems in my life or relationship, I continue to seek out and view pornography.

_____ Although it has caused problems in my life or relationship, I continue to masturbate.

_____ My spouse bullies me into having sex when I don't wish to.

_____ I (or my spouse) have been unfaithful.

_____ My spouse threatens that he (she) will have an affair if I don't agree to his (her) sexual demands.

_____ The sexual disagreements between my spouse and me are damaging the peace and harmony of our overall relationship.

_____ I am confronting a sexual issue I don't know how to handle effectively.

Additionally, counseling and other interventions (such as legal, social services) are always indicated in the following instances.

• If your spouse has sexual interests or habits that frighten you.

• If you or your spouse expresses sexual interest in children.

• If your spouse becomes physically violent during sex.

• If your spouse threatens to hurt you (or himself or herself) physically if you don't agree to sex.

WHERE TO TURN

While I have attempted to give you many tools you can use to work through basic disagreements, as well as principles that can be applied to evaluating the appropriateness of certain sexual practices, there can be times when you need to seek faithful counseling to help you resolve your struggles.

I can't emphasize enough the importance of seeking faithful solutions to your sexual problems. Matthew 8:36 asks the question, "What does it profit a man to gain the world but lose his soul?" It's important to work with a marital or sex counselor who can help you achieve your goals in a manner consistent with your faith so that you can become a truly Infallible Lover capable of enjoying the sensuality and *soulfulness* of Holy Sex. Counselors who don't understand your values may even *pathologize* certain aspects of your faith or moral principles. For instance, a secular counselor might tell you that all your sexual disagreements would be resolved if you'd simply stop using NFP, or agree to view pornography, or use masturbation as a way of learning to overcome premature ejaculation or anorgasmia. By contrast, counselors who are supportive of your faith and values are competent both clinically and theologically and can help you achieve the same goals a secular counselor would set for you (achieving a satisfying sexual relationship), but doing so using techniques that don't contradict your religious and moral principles.

In clinical practice, it is said that "ecological" solutions (that is, proposed changes that respect the client's values, responsibilities, and commitments) are the ones with the highest likelihood of working over the long haul. In fact, as research published in the *Journal of Counseling Psychology* demonstrates, religious clients have greater success in treatment when matched with therapists who share their values and use techniques that incorporate spiritual principles drawn from the client's faith.

Readers interested in applying the principles of their faith to overcoming sexual difficulties should seek out counselors who have the following qualifications. They should:

- have a master's degree or higher in a counseling-related discipline and be licensed at the highest level available in the state in which they practice;
- have theological training in addition to their clinical training and be both knowledgeable and supportive of Catholic teaching on sexual ethics;

- have specific knowledge about the practical applications of the Theology of the Body;

- be comfortable discussing sexual issues openly, and knowledgeable about conventional sex therapy treatments and how to adapt them for effective use with people of faith.

Admittedly, such counselors can be difficult to find. In 2005, the Pastoral Solutions Institute conducted a survey of religiously committed Catholics in all fifty states. The results of that study showed that respondents were overwhelmingly pessimistic about being able to find competent, faithful help in their area from either church or community-based mental health services. Faithful Catholics should not assume that counselors they are referred to by their pastor or diocese — or even those counselors directly employed by the Church — necessarily have the qualifications listed above. Clients are always responsible for evaluating the credentials of any counselor with whom they might work.

If you're unable to find local resources, the Pastoral Solutions Institute offers a full range of psychotherapeutic services (individual, marriage and parenting, and group) *via the telephone* to Catholics and other Christians worldwide. Pastoral Solutions counselors are licensed clinicians who also have advanced theological training. The Institute also has access to an advisory board of faithful theologians, clergy, canon lawyers, and Catholic physicians who can provide additional theological and clinical support for complex cases. Please feel free to contact us with any questions at (740) 266-6461 or online at *www.exceptionalmarriages.com*.

Though some may wonder about the effectiveness of counseling by telephone, in research published in flagship journals such as the *Archives of General Psychiatry* and the *Journal of Counseling Psychology*, among others, telecounseling has been shown to be as effective as face-to-face counseling for many types of problems. For example, according to research in the *Journal of Counseling and Development*, clients of telecounseling agencies actually found telecounseling *preferable* to face-to-face counseling — especially when dealing with sensitive issues where face-to-face contact might prove embarrassing. The Institute is an important resource for professionals who wish to learn more about practicing within a faith-integrated context, and those people of faith who are concerned about receiving care from a competent professional who is knowledgeable and supportive of their values.

BE NOT AFRAID

Regardless of where you ultimately turn to seek assistance, it is important to know that help is available, and the earlier you seek it, the more easily the issue will be resolved. Don't be afraid that your problem is too big, or not big enough. If you are struggling unsuccessfully with a particular issue in your sexual relationship, or your marriage as a whole, or if some personal problem is standing in the way of the joy God has willed for your life and relationships, reach out and trust that God has a faithful answer for you.

Be not afraid.

23 HOLY SEX IS YOUR INHERITANCE: GO IN PEACE

The most intense of pleasurable activities, I mean the passion of erotic love, is at the center of our focus so that we may learn that it is necessary for the soul, fixing itself steadily on the inaccessible beauty of divine nature, to love that nature as much as the body has a bent for what is akin to it, and to turn passion into impassibility, so that when every bodily disposition has been quelled, our mind within us may boil with love.

— St. Gregory of Nyssa, *On the Song of Songs*

Holy Sex is your inheritance. God gave sex to the godly, and it's time for us to take it back. Holy Sex is a sacred, redemptive, divine, uniting, and life-giving reality. It is real sex for real grown-ups. It is a celebration of all that is good in your marriage, and it is a means by which you draw the strength to make your marriage even better. As a sacrament, Holy Sex is an important part of the way God makes a couple perfect in love.

In this book, you have explored the traditional Christian view of sex. You have seen its power. You have witnessed its superiority to anything the world has to offer. You have discovered the lies and myths that are told to keep you from the fullness of Holy Sex, and you have identified faithful ways to solve the problems that seek to rob you of the joy that is yours.

All that is left is for you and your spouse to live the truth that sets you free. The family is the basis of society, and the foundation of the family is sex, for without it, there can be no family. By rescuing sex from those in the world who would hold it hostage, reclaiming it for Christ, and letting it challenge you to become the self-donative, generous lover God calls you to be in and out of the bedroom, you have the power to change the world because you have the power to create a healthy, joyful, loving family founded on authentic, incarnational, holy love.

Each time you and your spouse make love, you will say, "I do" all over again: not only to each other, but to God, who has asked you to love your mate as he himself loves your mate. Through Holy Sex, you will make the invisible reality of God's love for you and your love for each other visible and incarnate. Through Holy Sex, you and your spouse will discover and celebrate a passion that redeems you, sanctifies you, and enables you to rise in ecstasy toward the Divine. Through Holy Sex, you will find yourself in the authentic gift of yourself. Through Holy Sex, you will create the next generation of men and women who will build God's kingdom and live eternally in heaven.

Go in peace to love and to serve the Lord.

A WORD FROM THE AUTHOR

The Pastoral Solutions Institute
Faith-Filled Answers to Life's Toughest Questions
234 St. Joseph Drive
Steubenville, Ohio 43952
740-266-6461
www.ExceptionalMarriages.com

Marriage and family counseling agencies by their specific work of guidance and prevention... offer valuable help in rediscovering the meaning of love and life, and in supporting every family in its mission as the "sanctuary of life."

— Pope John Paul II, *The Gospel of Life*

Dear Friends,

I hope you've enjoyed this book, but everyone needs a little help from time to time. If you are struggling to apply your faith to your marriage, family, or personal and emotional problems, the Pastoral Solutions Institute tele-counseling services can help.

For many people, phone consultations provide just the right mix of professionalism, privacy, and convenience. Because you make the call from the comfort of your own home, sessions are completely confidential.

My associate counselors and I use a special clinical format that can help you begin to find solutions in our first session. You will end each phone contact with something new. A new technique, a new direction, more hope, greater resolve, and ultimately a tailor-made resolution. And because we utilize an advisory board of theologians, canon lawyers, physicians, and clergy, we can offer the most faithful and effective solutions to the problems you face. A simple phone call could be your first step on a journey to a more rewarding, more fulfilling life.

It's time to make a change for the better. Call or E-mail me today. Let Pastoral Solutions help you make your world a better place to live.

May God bless you abundantly,

Gregory K. Popcak, Ph.D., M.S.W.
Executive Director
Pastoral Solutions Institute

ABOUT THE AUTHOR

DR. GREGORY POPCAK (POP-chak) is a nationally recognized expert in pastoral counseling, especially in the areas of affective disorders (depression, anxiety) and marriage and family problems.

Greg earned a B.A. in Psychology and a B.A. in Theology from the University of Steubenville. He also holds an M.S.W. (Clinical Specialization) from the University of Pittsburgh and a Ph.D. in Human Services (with an emphasis in Pastoral Counseling) from Capella University. Additionally, he has received specific training in Functional Family Therapy at the Western Psychiatric Institute and Clinic, and Structural Family Therapy from the Philadelphia Child Guidance Institute.

Greg has conducted an active counseling practice — first face-to-face, and now telephonically — for over sixteen years. He is the founder/executive director of the Pastoral Solutions Institute, and the author of eight popular books integrating the Christian faith with counseling psychology. His articles and columns can regularly be found in publications such as *Catholic Parent, Family Foundations, Faith and Family, Our Sunday Visitor,* and others, and he has been interviewed on marriage and family issues in publications as diverse as *Columbia, Ladies' Home Journal,* and the *National Enquirer.*

He has hosted two television series for EWTN (*For Better . . . FOREVER!* and *God Help Me!*). Together with his wife, Lisa, Dr. Popcak hosts the daily nationally syndicated radio broadcast *Heart, Mind & Strength.*

Greg has been married to Lisa for sixteen years. The couple has three children, Jacob (fourteen), Rachel (twelve), and Liliana (nineteen months — adopted from China in March of 2007), who are homeschooled. Greg enjoys public speaking, writing, and, when he gets the chance, acting in community theater. The Popcak family lives in Steubenville, Ohio.

Of Related Interest

THE BAD CATHOLIC'S GUIDE TO GOOD LIVING

*A Loving Look at the Lighter Side of the Catholic Faith,
with Recipes for Feasts and Fun*

Text by John Zmirak and
recipes by Denise Matychowiak

Celebrate the Feast Days of the Saints — and don't forget your
trampoline!

Jump right into this hilarious book on enjoying and celebrating
Catholicism in a whole new way! Both a comical read and an indispensable resource for observing the Feast Days of the Saints,
The Bad Catholic's Guide to Good Living is for anyone interested
in celebrating the history and humor behind the Catholic Faith.
Consisting of selected monthly historical sketches of the feast
days, as well as suggested activities for celebration, this book
serves as a must-have for every happy Catholic! Written by
a Catholic journalist and a four-star chef, it's an entertaining
guide and guerilla catechism.

"Imagine Mel Gibson crossed with Monty Python — a hilarious,
in your face, Late-Nite Latin Mass."

— Angelo Matera, Publisher, Godspy.com,
former CEO of the *National Catholic Register*

0-8245-2300-8, paperback

crossroad

Of Related Interest

George William Rutler
COINCIDENTALLY

From the Da Vinci Code and Roswell to E Pluribus Unum and the pyramid on the back of every dollar bill, we all are fascinated by secrets, codes, and coincidences. George Rutler — EWTN speaker, *Crisis* magazine columnist, and reigning Catholic wit — offers his reflections on the coincidental links that connect the most far-flung parts of our worlds. Topics cover the gamut of human life, from Louis Farrakhan and Edgar Allan Poe to Benjamin Franklin and the propensity of Scottish physicians to dominate the Nobel Prizes for Medicine. Fr. George Rutler is best known as the host of a weekly program on EWTN and the pastor of Our Saviour in midtown New York City, where he lives.

0-8245-2440-3, hardcover

crossroad

Of Related Interest

John J. Dietzen
CATHOLIC Q & A
Answers to the Most Common Questions about Catholicism

Over 100,000 people have gone to their local Catholic book-store or parish to buy *Catholic Q & A*, the authoritative question and answer book from Fr. John J. Dietzen, columnist for the Catholic News Service. Crossroad is delighted to take over publication of this Guildhall Publishers classic.

Three features make this book unique. It is *comprehensive and current*. These hundreds of questions are drawn from real-life questions Fr. Dietzen has received over the years from readers and parishioners, and new questions are added for every edition to reflect current trends and issues. It is *Catholic*. Fr. Dietzen shows what the official church teaching is, as well as where church teaching is silent. It is *compassionate*. Fr. Dietzen writes with an engaging and warm pastoral style to convey the joy and wisdom of the Catholic faith.

Fr. John J. Dietzen has been a priest for over forty years and a columnist for the Catholic News Service since 1975. An earlier edition of this book won the Catholic Press Award for Popular Presentation of the Catholic Faith. Fr. Dietzen lives in Peoria, Illinois.

0-8245-2309-1, paper

crossroad

Of Related Interest

Pope Benedict XVI
THE YES OF JESUS CHRIST
Spiritual Exercises in Faith, Hope, and Love

Anyone wanting to understand Pope Benedict XVI's view of the relationship between Christianity and the world must read this eloquent book.

Secular thought has failed to answer the great questions of human existence. The "optimism" that lacks a Christian foundation ultimately cannot sustain genuine faith, hope, and love. In *The Yes of Jesus Christ,* Benedict XVI invites us to rediscover the Christian basis for hope. By exercising our spirituality through continual practice in Christian life, we hear again the distinctly Christian message that our ability to say Yes to ourselves and one another can only come from God's Yes in Christ.

Other Benedict XVI books available from Crossroad include *A New Song for the Lord: Faith in Christ and Liturgy Today* and *Values in a Time of Upheaval.*

0-8245-2374-1, paperback

Of Related Interest

Donna Marie Cooper O'Boyle
PRAYERFULLY EXPECTING
A Nine-Month Novena for Mothers to Be

Transform the traditional nine-day prayer of preparation for the great feast days into a nine-month devotional practice for your pregnancy. This keepsake prayer journal offers a place for an expecting mother to celebrate the mystery of pregnancy in prayer and reflection. Each part of the novena is accompanied with inspiring prayers, monthly updates about baby development, and supportive quotes from Blessed Mother Teresa of Calcutta, Pope John Paul II, and others. There is space for the expecting mother to collect personal prayers, reflections, and photos to be remembered for years to come.

0-8245-2450-4, paperback

crossroad

Of Related Interest

Joann Heaney-Hunter and Louis Primavera
UNITAS
Preparing for Sacramental Marriage

Based on the Rite of Christian Initiation for Adults, this marriage formation program is designed to help couples appreciate the importance of sacramental marriage in their lives and in the life of the wider church community.

Unitas Leader's Guide
0-8245-1755-5, paperback

Unitas Couples Workbook
0-8245-1756-3, paperback

Unitas Videotapes (set of 3)
0-8245-1757-1

Check your local bookstore for availability.
To order directly from the publisher,
please call 1-800-707-0670 for Customer Service
or visit our Web site at *www.cpcbooks.com.*
For catalog orders, please send your request to the address below.

THE CROSSROAD PUBLISHING COMPANY
16 Penn Plaza, Suite 1550
New York, NY 10001

crossroad